The Pain Ce...

Danielle Perret, MD
Assistant Dean for Resident Affairs
Director, Fellowship Program in Pain Medicine
Associate Director, Residency Training Program in
    Physical Medicine and Rehabilitation
Associate Clinical Professor
Department of Anesthesiology and Perioperative Care
Department of Physical Medicine and Rehabilitation
UCI Center for Pain Management
University of California-Irvine

Eric Chang, MD
Assistant Professor In-Residence
Division of Pain Medicine
Department of Anesthesiology and Perioperative Care
Department of Physical Medicine and Rehabilitation
Department of Orthopedics
Reeve-Irvine Research Center for Spinal Cord Injury
University of California-Irvine

Justin Hata, MD
Chief, Division of Pain Medicine
Director, Residency Training Program in Physical
    Medicine and Rehabilitation
Associate Clinical Professor
Department of Anesthesiology and Perioperative Care
Department of Physical Medicine and Rehabilitation
Medical Director
UCI Center for Pain Management
University of California-Irvine

Hamilton Chen, MD
Pain Medicine Fellow
Department of Anesthesiology and Perioperative Care
UCI Center for Pain Management
University of California-Irvine

Bianca Tribuzio, DO
Pain Medicine Fellow
Department of Physical Medicine and Rehabilitation
UCLA/West Los Angeles-VA

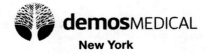

demosMEDICAL

New York

Visit our website at www.demosmedpub.com

ISBN: 9781620700211
e-book ISBN: 9781617051845

Acquisitions Editor: Beth Barry
Compositor: Exeter Premedia Services Private Ltd.

Medicine is an ever-changing science. Research and clinical experience are continually expanding our knowledge, in particular our understanding of proper treatment and drug therapy. The authors, editors, and publisher have made every effort to ensure that all information in this book is in accordance with the state of knowledge at the time of production of the book. Nevertheless, the authors, editors, and publisher are not responsible for errors or omissions or for any consequences from application of the information in this book and make no warranty, expressed or implied, with respect to the contents of the publication. Every reader should examine carefully the package inserts accompanying each drug and should carefully check whether the dosage schedules mentioned therein or the contraindications stated by the manufacturer differ from the statements made in this book. Such examination is particularly important with drugs that are either rarely used or have been newly released on the market.

Library of Congress Cataloging-in-Publication Data
Perret, Danielle, author.
The pain center manual / Danielle Perret, Eric Chang, Justin Hata, Hamilton Chen, Bianca Tribuzio
    p. ; cm.
  Includes bibliographical references.
  ISBN 978-1-62070-021-1—ISBN 978-1-61705-184-5 (e-book)
  I. Chang, Eric, author. II. Hata, Justin, author. III. Chen, Hamilton, author.
  IV. Tribuzio, Bianca, author. V. Title.
  [DNLM: 1. Pain Management—Handbooks. 2. Pain—drug therapy—Handbooks.
3. Pain Measurement—Handbooks. WL 39]
  RB127
  616'.0472—dc23

                                                                    2013033816

Special discounts on bulk quantities of Demos Medical Publishing books are available to corporations, professional associations, pharmaceutical companies, health care organizations, and other qualifying groups. For details, please contact:

Special Sales Department
Demos Medical Publishing, LLC
11 West 42nd Street, 15th Floor
New York, NY 10036
Phone: 800-532-8663 or 212-683-0072
Fax: 212-941-7842
E-mail: specialsales@demosmedpub.com

Printed in the United States of America by Gasch Printing.
13 14 15 16 17 / 5 4 3 2 1

Contents

Preface

Welcome to Pain Medicine done right. Patients in pain expect exceptionally qualified and compassionate care. Determining the appropriate approach for each patient is a nuanced art, but a solid grasp on the base knowledge can put this goal within reach.

This concise handbook is your continuous guide to the best practices reflective of academic pain management. It's not an encyclopedia, but it is full of pearls of knowledge for quick reference and on-the-spot training in both academic and community-based medicine. For the medical student or resident rotating through Pain, fellow in training, academic faculty, or private attending, this manual is your guide to our best practices. In these pages, you'll find common medication dosages, procedure templates, pharmacotherapies, and other useful diagnostic and treatment strategies, all reflective of interdisciplinary multimodal Pain Medicine techniques we use in the University of California chronic pain clinic and procedure suites. You'll also find a guide to the Accreditation Council for Graduate Medical Education (ACGME) standards, objectives, and suggested readings. Where large textbooks fail to offer practical guidelines for everyday pain management, this resource fills in the gaps.

This is the manual we rely on, every day, because it works. We hope it becomes a trusted resource for you as well.

Danielle Perret, MD
Assistant Dean for Resident Affairs
Director, Fellowship Program in Pain Medicine
Associate Director, Residency Training Program in
Physical Medicine and Rehabilitation
Associate Clinical Professor
Department of Anesthesiology and Perioperative Care
Department of Physical Medicine and Rehabilitation
UCI Center for Pain Management
University of California-Irvine

Opioids

Opioid Receptors

Mu: Midbrain, forebrain, cervicothoracic cord
Mu1 (*Morphine*): Supraspinal analgesia, bradycardia, sedation
Mu2: Respiratory depression, euphoria, physical dependence
Kappa (*Dynorphin, Nalbuphine, Butorphanol*): Weak spinal analgesia (lumbar spine), respiratory depression, sedation, inhibition of ADH, dyshporia, hallucinations
Delta (*Enkephalin*): Weak spinal analgesia (lumbar spine), respiratory depression; inhibits interneurons in the substantia gelatinosa causing GABA release
Sigma (*Pentazocine*): Dysphoria, delirium, mydriasis, hallucinations, tachycardia, HTN
Exogenous opioids act at: Periventricular area, PAG, rostroventral medulla

General Opioid Side Effects

- Increase in sphincter of Oddi tone; abnormal LFTs
- Constipation (dose dependent)
- Nausea and vomiting (medullary chemoreceptor trigger zone stimulation)
- *All opioid receptors are G-protein linked and cause*:
  - Presynaptic inhibition of neurotransmitters (Sub P, glutamate)
  - Postsynaptic inhibition of neurons by: opening K+ channels that hyperpolarize the cell

Tolerance

- Requires NMDA activation.
- *Tolerance* is selective; decreased risk with increased potency opioids; increased risk with benzodiazepines and with IV infusions versus PRN administration, reversible after 1 week, due to M3G metabolite.
- *NMDA antagonists* decrease the development of tolerance, potentiate opioid action, and decrease withdrawal symptoms.

Strategies to combat tolerance: Use higher potency opioids, use NMDA antagonists, coadminister alpha-2-agonist, coadminister NSAIDs, initiate opioid rotation, and simultaneously use opioids with different modes of action.

▓ SIGNS OF OPIOID WITHDRAWAL
Tachycardia, diaphoresis, nausea and vomiting, diarrhea, piloerection, insomnia, restlessness, tremor, fever, respiratory distress, increased mucus secretion, convulsions, facial scratching, pupillary dilation

▓ OPIOID OVERNARCOTIZATION
Nausea, vomiting, pruritus, pinpoint pupils, constipation, respiratory depression, urinary retention

▓ NOTES ON OPIOID ABUSE
Substance abuse in the United States = 7%
Most common illicit substance = marijuana
Most common abused substance = alcohol
Most common abused pain medication = Vicodin

Abuse increases in the United States with 4-year college education.

Largest nonmedical use of pain medications was between 1995 and 2000.

Simple detox (5 days) success = 2%–3%
6-month detox success = 65%
Mortality of substance abuser = 3×

DEA Class	Description	Examples
I	High abuse potential; no accepted medical use	Heroin, marijuana
II	High abuse potential; severe dependency (most narcotics)	Morphine, oxycodone, codeine, hydromorphone, hydrocodone, cocaine, amphetamines, methylphenidate, secobarbital
III	Moderate dependence liability	Vicodin, ketamine, buprenorphine, Tylenol #3
IV	Limited dependence liability	Propoxyphene, benzodiazepines,
V	Limited abuse potential but requires Rx	Lomotil

▓ OPIOID WITHDRAWAL PROTOCOL

ONSET/DURATION OF SYMPTOMS*

Starts <8 hr from opioid last use (peaks in 36–72 hr)	Anxiety, craving drug, lacrimation, chills, fear of withdrawal, diaphoresis, rhinorrhea, yawning
Starts 12 hr from opioid last use (peak in 72 hr)	Anxiety, restlessness, irritability, tremor, dysphoria, piloerection, anorexia, dilated pupils, abdominal cramps, mild tachycardia, and/or hypertension
Starts 24–36 hr from opioid last use (peak 72 hr)	Nausea, vomiting, diarrhea, abdominal cramps, myalgia, muscle spasms (especially in lower extremities), severe insomnia, violent yawning

*Methadone withdrawal may take longer to manifest clinically (24–48 hr from last dose) than withdrawal from other opioids, and may persist 2–3 weeks or longer.

CLINICAL FEATURES OF OPIOID WITHDRAWAL: DETECTED AND MONITORED USING OPIOID WITHDRAWAL SCALE (OWS)

Physical signs and symptoms*	Dilated pupils, diaphoresis, yawning, chills, piloerection, lacrimation, nausea, vomiting, abdominal cramps, diarrhea, rhinorrhea, mild tachycardia and/or hypertension

*Physical withdrawal symptoms generally resolve by 5–10 days.

Psychological symptoms**	Anxiety, restlessness, insomnia, fatigue, dysphoria, craving for opioids

**Psychological withdrawal symptoms (dysphoria, insomnia) may last weeks to months.

COMPLICATIONS OF OPIOID WITHDRAWAL

Opioid withdrawal is not life-threatening in healthy individuals.   – Need to continually assess all patients for suicide risk   – Screen for pregnancy   – Warn patients about overdose if they resume opioid at previous dose
Higher risk of complications in pregnant women and neonates   – Pregnancy-associated risks: spontaneous abortions, preterm labor   – Neonatal abstinence syndrome: seizure, death if not identified and treated
Serious risk of flight, suicide (precipitated by anxiety and dysphoria), and overdose on relapse because patients start to lose tolerance to opioids within 3–7 days after last use

Source: Adapted from Opioid Withdrawal Protocol by Peter Butt, MD, SCFP (EM), Melanie McLeod, BSP, ACPR, PharmD Candidate, and Christi Becker-Irvine, RN.

▨ OPIOID WITHDRAWAL PROTOCOL (*Continued*)

STEP 1: SYMPTOMATIC PROTOCOL AND CLONIDINE

SYMPTOMATIC PROTOCOL

Target Symptoms	Drugs	Dosing Guideline
Nausea and vomiting	Dimenhydrinate (Gravol)	50–100 mg PO (or IM) up to every 4 hr as needed
	Prochlorperazine (Stemetil)	5–10 mg PO up to every 4 hr as needed
	Loperamide (Imodium)	4 mg PO for diarrhea, then 2 mg PO as needed for loose bowel movements (max dose: 16 mg/24 hr)
Myalgia	Acetaminophen (Tylenol)	325–650 mg PO every 4 hr as needed (max dose: 3.5 g/24 hr)
	Naproxen (Naprosyn)	500 mg PO twice daily with meals for 4 days then reduce to twice daily as needed
Anxiety, dysphoria, lacrimation, rhinorrhea	Hydroxyzine (Atarax)	25–50 mg PO 3× daily as needed
Insomnia	Trazodone (Trazorel)	50–100 mg PO at bedtime × 4 days then as needed for insomnia

CLONIDINE

Dose	Monitoring
Clonidine 0.1 mg oral test dose	Check BP 1 hr later. If BP <90/60, if marked postural hypotension occurs, or if HR <60, do not prescribe further
If <91 kg (or <200 lb) – Clonidine 0.1 mg PO 4× a day for 4 days – Clonidine 0.05 mg PO 4× a day for 2 days – Clonidine 0.025 mg PO 4× a day for 2 days, then stop	Check BP prior to each dose and withhold dose if BP <90/60, if marked postural hypotension or dizziness occurs or if HR <60 Assess Opioid Withdrawal Score (OWS) at least every 24 hr
If >91 kg (or >200 lb) – Clonidine 0.2 mg PO 4× day for 4 days – Clonidine 0.1 mg PO 4× a day for 2 days – Clonidine 0.05 mg PO 4× a day × 2 days – Clonidine 0.025 mg PO 4× a day × 1 day	If after 24 hr the OWS is 10–14 (suggesting moderate withdrawal symptoms), proceed to step 2 If after 24 hr, the OWS is >15 (suggesting severe withdrawal symptoms), proceed to step 3

Source: Adapted from Opioid Withdrawal Protocol by Peter Butt, MD, SCFP (EM), Melanie McLeod, BSP, ACPR, PharmD Candidate, and Christi Becker-Irvine, RN.

■ OPIOID WITHDRAWAL PROTOCOL *(Continued)*

STEP 2: SYMPTOMATIC PROTOCOL + INTENSIFIED CLONIDINE

Clonidine Dose	Monitoring
If <91 kg (or <200 lb) – Clonidine 0.2 mg PO 4× a day × 4 days – Clonidine 0.1 mg PO 4× a day × 2 days – Clonidine 0.05 mg PO 4× a day × 1 day – Clonidine 0.025 mg PO 4× a day × 1 day	Check BP prior to each dose and withhold dose if BP is <90/60, if marked postural hypotension or dizziness occurs, or if HR is <60 Assess Opioid Withdrawal Score (OWS) at least every 24 hr
If >91 kg (or >200 lb) – Clonidine 0.3 mg PO 4× a day × 4 days – Clonidine 0.2 mg PO 4× a day × 1 day – Clonidine 0.2 mg PO 4× a day × 1 day – Clonidine 0.05 mg PO 4× a day × 1 day – Clonidine 0.025 mg PO 4× a day × 1 day	If after 24 hr at step 2, the OWS is >15 (suggesting severe withdrawal symptoms) proceed to step 3

STEP 3: SYMPTOMATIC PROTOCOL + INTENSIFIED CLONIDINE + PHENOBARBITAL

Clonidine Dose	Monitoring
If <91 kg (or <200 lb) – Clonidine 0.2 mg PO 4× a day × 4 days – Clonidine 0.1 mg PO 4× a day × 2 days – Clonidine 0.05 mg PO 4× a day × 1 day – Clonidine 0.025 mg PO 4× a day × 1 day, then stop	Check BP prior to each dose and withhold dose if BP <90/60, if marked postural hypotension or dizziness occurs, or if HR <60 Assess Opioid Withdrawal Score (OWS) at least every 24 hr
If >91 kg (or >200 lb) – Clonidine 0.3 mg PO 4× a day × 4 days – Clonidine 0.2 mg PO 4× a day × 1 day – Clonidine 0.1 mg PO 4× a day × 1 day – Clonidine 0.05 mg PO 4× a day × 1 day – Clonidine 0.025 mg PO 4× a day × 1 day, then stop	

Phenobarbital Dose	Monitoring
Phenobarbital 30–60 mg PO twice daily as needed for anxiety and sedation	Hold dose in presence of marked sedation, hypotension (BP <90/60), dizziness, ataxia, listlessness. Stop if rash develops

▨ OPIOID WITHDRAWAL PROTOCOL (*Continued*)

STEP 4: REFER TO METHADONE PRESCRIBING PHYSICIAN

Methadone Dose	Monitoring
*Methadone 10 mg PO 3 times a day for 3–4 days Taper by 10 mg/day (5 mg/day on final dose)	Methadone-related deaths have occurred almost exclusively at dose in excess of 30 mg/day
*Alternatively, start at lower dose and titrate up to 30 mg/day.	

Source: Adapted by Opioid Withdrawal Protocol by Dr. Peter Butt, MD, SCFP (EM); Melanie McLeod BSP, ACPR, PharmD Candidate; Christi Becker-Irvine RN.

▩ OPIOID SCREENING TOOLS:
SOAPP® VERSION 1.0–14Q

Name: _____ Date: _____

The following are some questions given to all patients at Pain Management Center who are on or being considered for opioids for their pain. Please answer each question as honestly as possible. This information is for our records and will remain confidencial. Your answers alone will not determine your treatment. Thank you.

Please answer the questions below using the following scale

0 = Never, 1 = Seldome, 2 = Sometimes, 3 = Often, 4 = Very often

1. How often do you have mood swings?	0 1 2 3 4
2. How often do you smoke a cigarette within an hour after you wake up?	0 1 2 3 4
3. How often have any of your family members, including parents and grandparents, had a problem with alcohol or drugs?	0 1 2 3 4
4. How often have any of your close friends had a problem with alcohol or drugs?	0 1 2 3 4
5. How often have others suggested that you have a drug or alcohol problem?	0 1 2 3 4
6. How often have you attended ar. AA or NA meeting?	0 1 2 3 4
7. How often have you taken medication other than the way that it was prescribed?	0 1 2 3 4
8. How often have you been treated for an alcohol or drug problem?	0 1 2 3 4
9. How often have your medications been lost or stolen?	0 1 2 3 4
10. How often have others expressed concern over your use of medication?	0 1 2 3 4
11. How often have you fells a craving for medicaton?	0 1 2 3 4
12. How often have you been asked to give a urine screen for substance abuse?	0 1 2 3 4
13. How often have you used illegal drugs (for example, marijuana, cocaine, etc.) in the past five years?	0 1 2 3 4
14. How often in your lifetime have you had legal problems or been arrested?	0 1 2 3 4

SOAPP® Version 1.0–14Q (Continued)

To score the SOAPP® Version 1.0–14Q, simply add the ratings of all the questions: A score of 7 or higher is considered positive.

Sum of Questions	SOAPP® Indication
> or = 7	+
> 7	–

SOAPP® cutoff score	Sensitivity	Specificity	Positive predictive value	Negative predictive value	Positive likelihood ratio	Negative likelihood ratio
Score 7 or above	.91	.69	.71	.90	2.94	.13
Score 8 or above	.86	.73	.75	.86	3.19	.19
Score 9 or above	.77	.80	.77	.80	3.90	.28

OPIOID RISK TOOL

		Mark each box that applies	Item score if female	Item score if male
1. Family history of substance abuse	Alcohol	[ ]	1	3
	Illegal drugs	[ ]	2	3
	Prescription drugs	[ ]	4	4
2. Personal history of substance abuse	Alcohol	[ ]	3	3
	Illegal drugs	[ ]	4	4
	Prescriptioon drugs	[ ]	5	5
3. Age (Mark box if 16–45)		[ ]	1	1
4. History of preadolescent sexual abuse		[ ]	3	0
5. Psychological disease	Attention deficit disorder	[ ]	2	2
	Obsessive compulsive disorder			
	Bipolar schizophrenia			
	Depression	[ ]	1	1
Total		[ ]		
Total score risk category	Low risk 0–3	Moderate risk 4–7	High risk ≥ 8	

Source: Reproduced with permission from Lynn Webster.

Narcotic Conversions

```
100 mcg IV fentanyl =
1 mg epidural morphine =
0.1 mg intrathecal morphine =
30 mg PO morphine = (3:1 PO:IV)
30 mg PO hydrocodone =
20 mg PO oxycodone = (3:2 oxycodone:morphine)
200 mg PO codeine = (10:1 oxycodone:codeine)
7.5 mg PO hydromorphone = (5:1 hydromorphone:morphine)
1.5 mg IV hydromorphone = (1:5 PO:IV)
30 mg PO morphine = 300 mg PO Demerol = 75 mg IV Demerol
```

Source: Analgesics. *Tarascon Pocket Pharmacopoeia* 2008.

NARCAN INFUSION
2–4 mg/500 mL D5W or NS
Run at 0.4 mg/hr = 100 mL/hr
Ampules contain 1 mL = 0.4 mg
Administer 0.04 mg (40 mcg) = 1 ampule diluted in 10 mL NS (increments at 2-min intervals)
Side effects: pulmonary edema, seizures, V-fib, and cardiac arrest

Source: Reversal Agents, Complications in Anesthesia. *Expert Consult* and http://www.druglib.com

MORPHINE IT TRIALS
500 mcg bolus: If no response, increase bolus by 2×; and so forth.
Response = 50% reduction in pain for at least 2× the narcotic half-life (8–12 hr for morphine)
Must stop long-acting opioids.
Also FDA approved: Baclofen and Ziconotide (Prialt = CCB)

FENTANYL
Max dose = 300 mcg (patch)
Half-life = 17 hr

Fentanyl	PO Morphine	IV Morphine
25 mcg	45–134 mg/day	8–22 mg/day
50 mcg	135–224 mg/day	23–37 mg/day
75 mcg	225–314 mg/day	38–52 mg/day
100 mcg	315–404 mg/day	53–67 mg/day

Source: Pain, Chronic Pain. *Tarascon Primary Care Pocketbook* 2010.

Fentanyl Safety:
Write date and time on patch.
Put over muscle or fatty tissue.

Methadone

▉ SAFETY CONSIDERATIONS

Interpatient variability in the drug's absorption, metabolism, and relative analgesic potency necessitates a highly individualized approach to prescribing with particular vigilance during treatment initiation and titration.

Incomplete cross-tolerance between methadone and other opioids makes dosing during opioid conversion complex. A high degree of tolerance to other opioids does not eliminate the possibility of methadone overdose.

While methadone's duration of analgesic action for single doses (4–8 hr) approximates that of morphine, the drug's half-life is substantially longer than that of morphine (8–59 hr vs. 1–5 hr).

With chronic use, methadone may be retained in the liver and then slowly released, prolonging the duration of action despite low plasma concentrations.

Due to the long half-life, full analgesic effects may not be attained until after 3–5 days of use; thus, the drug must be titrated more slowly than other opioids.

Methadone's peak respiratory depressant effects typically occur later and persist longer than its peak analgesic effects.

If methadone is not taken for 3 consecutive days, the patient may lose tolerance to methadone and be at risk for an overdose if the usual dose is taken.

▓ PRESCRIBING METHADONE

Evaluate the patient's risk of abusing the drug and his/her ability to comply with methadone's administration directions. Consider alternative pain medications if the patient is deemed to be at risk.

Designate all patients as opioid-naive for the purposes of introducing methadone, no matter how much opioid medication they've previously been taking. To start with, consider a conservative ceiling dose of no more than 20 mg/day (10 mg/day for elderly/infirm).

Do not adjust doses more often than weekly.

Allow a steady state of methadone plasma levels to develop and evaluate patients for untoward effects before titrating the dose upward. Be sure to ask patients about adverse effects before increasing the dose.

Prescribe oral liquid doses of methadone in mg, never in mL alone, since several concentrations exist. Include the indication for use when prescribing methadone: FOR PAIN.

Specify the exact time(s) for administration; every 8 hr, NOT three times a day. Even daily doses, if taken in the evening one day and in the morning the next day, can lead to overdose.

Avoid concomitant use of methadone with other narcotics, benzodiazepines, and sedatives, as these significantly increase the risk of an adverse event.

If patients must take these medications concomitantly, the starting dose and speed of titration for methadone may need to be adjusted downward.

Closely monitor patients.

▓ METHADONE RISK FACTORS

QTc interval >500 ms

QTc interval 451–500 mg

Family history of: long QT syndrome, early sudden cardiac death, or electrolyte depletion

Concomitant therapy with a cytochrome P450 inhibitor

Concomitant therapy/use of other QTc interval-prolonging drug

Concomitant use of a benzodiazepine

History of psychiatric admission

History of unexplained generalized seizure

History of unexplained syncope

History of structural heart disease, arrhythmia, or previous myocardial infarction

History of hepatic disease, malnutrition, electrolyte abnormalities, or hypokalemia

Methadone use >100 mg/day

IV (vs. PO) methadone use

History of noncompliance in patient record

Increase in QTc interval by >10 ms from baseline since initiation of methadone therapy

Concomitant use of another opioid medication

P450 Inhibitors

Acitretin
Amiodarone
Amprenavir
Aprepitant
Atazanavir
Bupropion
Celecoxib
Chloroquine
Chlorpheniramine
Cimetidine
Cinacalcet
Ciprofloxacin
Citalopram
Clarithromycin
Clomipramine
Cocaine
Cyclosporine
Danazol
Darifenacin
Delavirdine
Desipramine
Diltiazem
Diethyl-dithiocarbamate
Diphenhydramine
Duloxetine
Echinacea
Efavirenz
Enoxacin
Erythromycin
Escitalopram
Ethinyl

Estradiol
Fluconazole
Fluoxetine
Fluphenazine
Fluvoxamine
Gestodene
Grapefruit
Halofantrine
Haloperidol
Hydroxychloroquine
Imatinib
Indinavir
Isoniazid
Itraconazole
Ketoconazole
Levomepromazine
Methoxsalen
Metronidazole
Methylprednisolone
Mexiletine
Miconazole
Mifepristone
Nalidixic Acid
Moclobemide
Nefazodone
Nelfinavir
Nicardipine
Nifedipine
Norfluoxetine
Norethindrone
Norfloxacin

Omeprazole
Oral contraceptives
Oxiconazole
Paroxetine
Perphenazine
Pomegranate
Prednisone
Propafenone
Propoxyphene
Propanolol
Quinacrine
Quinidine
Quinine
Ranitidine
Ranolazine
Ritonavir
Roxithromycin
Saquinavir
Sertraline
Syncercid
Tacrine
Telithromycin
Terbinafine
Thioridazine
Ticlopidine
Tipranavir
Troleandomycin
Verapamil
Voriconazole
Zafirlukast
Zileuton

QT Prolonging Drugs

Alfuzosin
Amantidine
Amiodarone
Amitriptyline
Aresenic trioxide
Asternizole
Atazanavir
Azithromycin
Bepridil
Chloral hydrate
Chlorpromazine
Chloroquine
Ciprofloxacin
Cisapride
Citalopram
Clarithromycin
Clomipramine
Clozapine
Desipramine
Diphenhydramine
Disopyramide
Dofetilide
Dolasetron
Domperidone
Doxepin
Droperidol
Erythromycin
Felbamate
Flecainide
Fluconazole

Fluoxetine
Foscarnet
Fosphenytoin
Galantamine
Gatifloxacin
Gemifloxacin
Granisetron
Halofantrine
Haloperidol
Ibutilide
Imipramine
Indapamide
Isradipine
Itraconazole
Ketoconazole
Lithium
Levomethadyl
Mesoridazine
Methadone
Mexiletine
Moexipril/HCTZ
Moxifloxacin
Nicardipine
Nilotinib
Nortriptyline
Octreotide
Ofloxacin
Ondansetron
Oxytocin
Papileridone

Paroxetine
Pentamidine
Perflutren
Pimozide
Probuco
Procainamide
Protriptyline
Quetiapine
Quinidine
Ranolazine
Risperidone
Roxithromycin
Sertindole
Sertraline
Solifenacin
Sotalol
Sparfloxacin
Sunitinib
Tacrolimus
Tamoxifen
Telithromycin
Terfenadine
Thioridazine
Tizanidine
Trimethoprim sulfa
Trimipramine
Vardenafil
Venlfaxine
Voriconazole
Ziprasidon

Urine Drug Toxicity (UDT) Screens

▨ INTERPRETATION OF URINE TOXICITY RESULTS

Urine testing is most widely used because it is noninvasive, simple to obtain, and yields a detectable concentration of most drugs. False positives and false negatives exist. Immunoassays are used to screen; more specific gas chromatography mass spectrometry (GC/MS) can be performed for specific drugs.

Opioids (overview): In general, synthetic opioids such as fentanyl, Dilaudid, methadone, and meperidine are not picked up in standard screen and require specific tests (GC/MS). However codeine, morphine, and heroin are natural opioids and are generally found in screens.

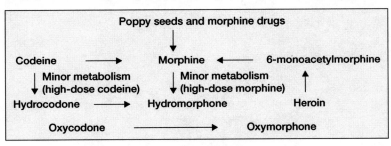

Common Interpretation Error 1: Patient on oxycodone and "none detected" on opioid screen. Patient accused of nonadherence because GC/MS not performed. *Solution:* Must perform GC/MS specific for oxycodone. Of note, oxycodone can metabolize to oxymorphone, so both may be seen.

Common Interpretation Error 2: Patient on hydrocodone, urine screen positive. GC/MS confirms hydrocodone and hydromorphone. Patient accused of misuse. *Solution:* Must understand drug metabolism as noted on the chart above.

Medical explanation of positive codeine result: Codeine is metabolized to morphine so prescribed codeine can explain the presence of both drugs in urine (though prescribed codeine should not explain ONLY morphine). Prescribed codeine may explain a trace of hydrocodone.

Medical explanation of positive cocaine result: Usually positive for 2–3 days. Occasionally used in dental, trauma, and ENT cases but otherwise cocaine is NOT falsely positive from any other "-caine" drugs or herbal teas.

Compiled by Justin Busch, MD.

Medical explanation of positive amphetamine/methamphetamine result: Prescription ADD drugs, many Parkinson's/decongestant medications (dopamine, ephedrine, phentermine, etc.) may yield a positive result. Some drugs are metabolized to amphetamines such as selegiline, benzphetamine, and a few others and may yield a positive result. Amphetamines exist as two isomers and separation of these isomers can help elucidate the medication behind a positive test.

Remember, negative UDT can mean ANY of the following: The patient has not used a drug, the patient has not recently used a drug, the patient excretes/metabolizes a drug more rapidly than normal, or the drug is present but in a concentration lower than detection level!

Urine Drug Toxicity (UDT) Screens (Continued)

▧ TYPES OF UDT

1. *Thin layer chromatography*: Old technique tests against a known control, $

2. *Enzyme immunoassay*: More sensitive than TLL, cost $$, uses antibodies

3. *Gas chromotography*: Most sensitive and specific, most reliable, labor intensive, $$$, takes several days

Amphetamine/methamphetamines are highly cross-reactive and not specific (other sympathomimetics will be detected such as ephedrine): further testing is required.

Tests for opiates are very responsive for morphine and codeine but poor at distinguishing between them (EIA).

UDTs have a low sensitivity for synthetic or semisynthetic opioids such as oxycodone (order gas chromatography).

A negative response does not exclude oxycodone/methadone use.

Marinol/protonix may test marijuana positive.

Duration

EtoH: 3–5 days via ethyl glucuronide
EtoH: 10–12 hr via traditional test

Amphetamine	1–2d
Methamphet	2–4d
Barbituates	2–3d
Benzos	3d
Benzos (chronic)	4–6w
Cocaine	2–4d
Codeine	1d
Cotinine (Nicotine)	2–4d
Morphine	2d
Methadone	3d
LSD	2–24h
Heroin	2d
Heroin (chronic)	2–5d
Phenobarb	1–2w
PCP	1–2w
Cannabis	1w
Cannabis (chronic)	1–3m

Controlled Substance Rx Writing Skills

UC Irvine Multispecialty Clinic
Gottschalk Medical Plaza; Irvine, CA 92697-6250
(949) 824-8600

UC Irvine
Healthcare

000152

☑ Danielle Perret
Dept. of Anesthesiology/Pain Management

SECURITY FEATURES LISTED ON BACK

PATIENT NAME: *Doe, Jane*
ADDRESS:
DOB: *1-1-34*
PH. NO.:
GENDER: *Fe*

1) *Methadone 10mg* *#90*
T tab po Q8h for pain

Quantity: ☐ 1-24 ☐ 25-49 ☐ 50-74 ☒ 75-100
☐ 101-150 ☐ 151-over Unit *90*
Refills: ⓪ · 1 · 2 · 3 · 4 · 5
☐ Do Not Substitute
Dispense As: ☐ First Time ☐ Refill

2)

Quantity: ☐ 1-24 ☐ 25-49 ☐ 50-74 ☐ 75-100
☐ 101-150 ☐ 151-over Unit
Refills: 0 · 1 · 2 · 3 · 4 · 5
☐ Do Not Substitute Initials
Dispense As: ☐ First Time Fill ☐ Refill

3)

Quantity: ☐ 1-24 ☐ 25-49 ☐ 50-74 ☐ 75-100
☐ 101-150 ☐ 151-over Unit
Refills: 0 · 1 · 2 · 3 · 4 · 5
☐ Do Not Substitute Initials
Dispense As: ☐ First Time Fill ☐ Refill

Signature _____ Date *4/20/08*

Prescription is void if the number of drugs is not noted: *ONE*
BLUE BACKGROUND. REFLECTIVE WATERMARK ON BACK.

Cross out boxes not used.

Re-write the number of tablets dispensed under "units."

Don't forget to tally the number of medications dispensed at the bottom. Otherwise, the Rx is void.

Check the correct box to specify the number of tablets dispensed for each medication.

Methadone should always be written with the words: "for pain" unless it is being prescribed for addiction; in that case an addiction medicine license is needed.

Controlled Substance Rx Sample

Cross out boxes not used.

Indicate the number of tablets dispensed.

Don't forget to tally the number of medications dispensed.

Check the appropriate box to specify the number of tablets dispensed.

Circle refills, if given. Controlled substances cannot be refilled, however.

Drug Names	Receptors	Mechanism	Side Effects	Overdose Information	Treatment
TCA amitryptiline, imipramine, trimipramine, nortyrptyline, desipramine	H2, alpha-1, muscarinic, and SNRI activity	Blockade of H2, blockade of alpha-1, and blockade of muscarinic receptors, as well as SNRI activity (see below)	Decreased gastric acid secretion (anti H2); orthostatic hypotension (anti alpha-1); constipation, tachycardia, blurry vision, urinary retention (anti-muscarinic)	Coma, prolonged QT; SVT; severe hypotension, seizure	Supportive care, physostigmine (watch for bradycardia), lidocaine, bicarbonate, potassium, diazepam (for seizure), transcutaneous pacing
SNRI venlafaxine, duloxetine, desvenlafaxine (tramadol, methadone, ketamine, TCAs have SNRI activity)	5-HT, adrenergic	Inhibit reuptake of the neurotransmitters serotonin and norepinephrine	Loss of appetite, weight loss, sleep disturbances, dizziness, HA, n/v, sexual dysfunction, urinary retention	Often due to combining with other antidepressants. Somnolence, coma, serotonin syndrome, seizure, tachycardia, hypotension, hypertension	Supportive care, cyproheptadine for serotonin syndrome
NMDA antagonists Ketamine (NMDA antag, SNRI activity, muscarinic activity), methadone (muagonism, NMDA antag), dextromethorphan	NMDA	Blockade of NMDA receptor, which are calcium-permeable ion channel that requires both glutamate and glycine for activation	Ketamine: analgesia, dissociation, sympathetic stimulation, minimal respiratory effects	Ketamine: sedation, respiratory arrest, hallucinations, dissociation, increased HR, HTN, blurry vision, seizures	Supportive care, benzodiazepines for seizure

(Continued)

COMMON MEDICATIONS USED IN PAIN MANAGEMENT (*Continued*)

Drug Names	Receptors	Mechanism	Side Effects	Overdose Information	Treatment
Sodium channel blockers (local anesthetics)					
Lidocaine, Bupivicaine, Ropivicaine, Tetracaine, Procaine	Sodium channels in neuronal cell membrane (voltage gated Na channels)	The drug is a weak base, traverses cell membrane in unionized form, becomes ionized inside cell, and binds to the cytoplasmic-facing site of receptor	Nerve damage, hypotension (rare), nausea (rare)	Arrhythmia, cardiac arrest, methemoglobinemia	Supportive care, intralipid to bind free LA
Substance P inhibitors					
Capsaicin	Neurokinin-1	Affects synthesis, storage, and release of substance P. Prevents reaccumulation of substance P in joints. Reduction in TRPV-expressing nociceptive nerve endings	Erythema of application site, nausea, nasopharyngitis, HTN	Rarely HTN	Supportive care, wash off skin
Alpha-2 agonists					
Clonidine, Tizanidine	Alpha-2 adrenergic	Agonist of presynaptic alpha-2 receptor, decreasing presynaptic calcium levels and decreasing release of NE	Lightheadedness, dry mouth, dizziness, constipation, hypotension (clonidine), rebound HTN (clonidine)	Hypotension, HTN, CNS depression, drowsiness, decreased RR, coma, seizure	Supportive care, can consider pumping stomach

(*Continued*)

COMMON MEDICATIONS USED IN PAIN MANAGEMENT (*Continued*)

Drug Names	Receptors	Mechanism	Side Effects	Overdose Information	Treatment
Opioids Morphine, Hydrocodone, Hydromorphone, Fentanyl, oxycodone	Mu, kappa, delta	Bind opioid receptors. Delta = analgesia, antidepressant, dependence. Kappa = analgesia, sedation, dysphoria. Mu = analgesia, dependence, respiratory depression, miosis, reduced GI motility	n/v, drowsiness, constipation (no tolerance to this problem), itching, dry mouth, miosis, hallucinations	Delirium, decreased consciousness, hypotension, respiratory depression	Naloxone, supportive care
Calcium channel blockers (antiepileptics) Gabapentin, Pregabalin, Ziconotide	L type calcium channels	Complex, much is unknown. Thought to bind to alpha-2 delta subunit of voltage dependent L-type calcium channels	Dizziness, fatigue, weight gain, drowsiness, peripheral edema, mood swings	Lethargy, difficulty breathing, hepatotoxicity	Supportive care, can consider dialysis
Sodium channel blockers (antiepileptics) Carbamazepine, Valproate, Lamotrigine, Oxcarbamazepine, Topiramate	Sodium channels in neuronal cell membrane (voltage-gated sodium channels)	Stabilizes the inactivated state of voltage-gated sodium channels, making fewer of these channels available to open. Leaves affected cells less excitable	n/v, abdominal pain, weight disturbances, dizziness, nystagmus, HA, tremor	CNS depression, hepatic failure, pancreatitis, tachycardia, seizure, shock, coma	Supportive care, proemetics, diuretics can be considered

Compiled by Justin Busch, MD.

Suggested Outpatient Medication Prescriptions

Antispasmodic
Baclofen 10 mg; ½ tablet tid; #45
Baclofen 10 mg; 1 tablet tid; #90
Flexeril 10 mg; ½ tablet Q8h; #45
Skelaxin 800 mg; 1 tablet tid; #90
Skelaxin 800 mg; 1 tablet qid; #120
Valium 2 mg; 1–2 tablets prior to procedure; #2
Zanaflex 2 mg; 1 tablet tid; #90
Zanaflex 4 mg; 1 tablet tid; #90
Zanaflex 6 mg; 1 tablet tid; #90

Nonsteroidal Anti-inflammatory
Celebrex 200 mg; 1 tablet bid; #60
Diclofenac 50 mg; 1 tablet tid; #90
Flector patch 180 mg; 1 patch daily; #30
Mobic 7.5 mg; 1 tablet daily; #30
Mobic 15 mg; 1 tablet daily; #30
Motrin 400 mg; 1 tablet tid; max 1.2 g/day #90
Naprosyn 500 mg; 1 tablet bid; #60

Neuropathic
Cymbalta 30 mg; 1 tablet qday; #30
Cymbalta 30 mg; 1 tablet bid; #60
Cymbalta 60 mg; 1 tablet qday; #30
Cymbalta 60 mg; 1 tablet bid; #60
Effexor XR 37.5/75 mg; 1 tablet qday; #30
Lyrica 75 mg; 1 tablet bid; #60
Lyrica 150 mg; 1 tablet bid; #60
Lyrica 50 mg; 1 tablet tid; #90
Lyrica 100 mg; 1 tablet tid; #90
Neurontin 100 mg; 3 capsules tid; #270 (see titration schedule)
Neurontin 300/400 mg; 1–3 capsules tid; max 3600 mg/day; #90–270
Neurontin oral solution 250 mg/5 mL; 2.5–5–10 mL tid; #470 mL bottle
Tegretol 100 mg; 1 tablet bid with food; #60
Tegretol 200 mg; 1 tablet bid with food; #60
Tegretol 400 mg; 1 tablet bid with food; #60

---

*Lamictal, Tegretol, Topamax: see also titration schedules on pp. 29–30.

Suggested Outpatient Medication Prescriptions (Continued)

Neuropathic
Lidoderm patch 5%; 1–2 patches daily for 12 hr applied; #30–60

Catapres TTS-1; 1 patch q7d; #4

Capsaicin 0.025%, 0.075% cream; apply tid–qid.

Weak Opioids
Ultram 50 mg; 1 tablet bid; #60
Ultram 50 mg; 1 tablet tid; #90
Ultram 50 mg: 1–2 tablets tid; #180

Ultram ER 100 mg; 1 tablet qday; #30
Ultram ER 200 mg; 1 tablet qday; #30
Ultram ER 300 mg; 1 tablet qday; #30

Migraine Prophylaxis
Naprosyn 500 mg; 1 tablet bid; #60

Propanolol 20 mg; 1 tablet qid; #120

Topamax 25 mg; 1 tablet qhs; #30
Topamax 25 mg; 1 tablet bid; #60
Topamax 25 mg; 1 qam; 2 tablets qhs; #90
Topamax 50 mg; 1 tablet bid; #60

Migraine Acute Treatment
Imitrex 25 mg; 1–3 tablets qHA; may repeat once after 2 hr; max 200 mg/day; #9
Imitrex Nasal Spray 5 mg; 1 qHA; may repeat once after 2 hr; max 40 mg/day; #6 bottles

Maxalt 5 mg; 1–2 tablets qHA; may repeat once after 2 hr; max 15 mg/day; #6

Zomig 2.5 mg; ½–1 tablet qHA; may repeat after 2 hr; max 10 mg/day; #6
Zomig Nasal Spray 5 mg; 1 qHA; may repeat once after 2 hr; max 10 mg/day; #6 bottles

Suggested Outpatient Medication Prescriptions (Continued)

Bone Pain
Miacalcin 200 units/spray; 1 spray to alternating nostrils q day; # 3.7 mL

Short-Acting Opioids
Dilaudid 2/4/8 mg; 1 tablet tid–qid PRN; #90–120

Fentora 100 mcg; 1 buccal tablet q4h PRN; #28
Fentora 200/400/600/800 mcg; 1 buccal tablet q4h PRN; #28

Morphine Sulfate IR 15/30 mg; 1 tablet q4–8h PRN; #90–180

Norco [5 mg HC/325 mg acetaminophen]; 1 tablet q4–8h PRN; max 8 tablets/day; #90–180
Norco [5/325] mg; 1–2 tablets q4–8h PRN; max 8 tablets/day; #240
Norco [10/325] mg

Nucynta (Tapentadol) [50/75/100 mg] 1 tablet Q4h #180

Opana (Oxymorphone) 5/10 mg; 1 tablet q4–6h PRN; #120–180

Oxy IR 5 mg; 1 tablet q4–8h PRN; #90–180
Oxy IR 5 mg; 2–3 tablets q4–8h PRN; #180–360 (#270–540)

Percocet 5 mg oxycodone/325 mg Acetaminophen; 1–2 tablets q4–6h PRN; max 10 tablets/day; #300
Percocet [10/325]/[7.5/325] mg; 1–2 tablets q4–6h PRN; max 10 tablets/day; #300
Percocet [7.5/500] mg; 1 tablet q4h PRN; max 6 tablets/day; #180
Percocet [10/650] mg; 1 tablet q4h PRN; max 5 tablets/day; #150

Roxicet Oral Solution (Oxy 5 mg/Tylenol 325 mg/5 mL); 5 mL q4–6h PRN; max 50 mL/day; #500 mL

Roxanol = Morphine Sulfate IR Oral Solution 20 mg/5 mL; 5 mL q4h PRN; #120 mL

Tylenol #3 (Codeine) [30/300] mg; 1–2 tablets q4h PRN; max 10 tablets/day; #300
Tylenol Codeine Elixir (Codeine 12 mg/120 mg/5 mL); 15 mL q4h PRN; max 125 mL/day; #1 pt

Vicodin [5 mg HC/500] mg; 1–2 tablets q4–6h PRN; max 6 tablets/day; #180
Vicodin ES [7.5 mg HC/750] mg; 1 tablet q6h PRN; max 4 tablets/day; #120

Suggested Outpatient Medication Prescriptions (Continued)

Long-Acting Opioids
Avinza (Morphine ER+ portions IR) 30/60/90 mg qday; max 1.6 g/day; #30

Duragesic (Fentanyl) 12/25/50/75/100 mcg; 1 patch q72h or q48h; #10

Exalgo (hydromorphone ER) 8/12/16/32 mg; 1 tablet q24h #30

Kadian (Morphine ER may sprinkle on applesauce)
10/20/30/50/60/80/100/200 mg; 1 tablet q12–24h; #30–60

MS Contin (Morphine CR) 15/30/60/100/200 mg; 1 tablet bid–tid; #60–90

Nucynta ER (Tapentadol) [50/100/150/200/250 mg] 1 tablet Q12h #60

Opana ER (Oxymorphone ER) 5/7.5/10/15/20/30/40 mg; 1 tablet q12h

Oxycontin (oxycodone CR) 10/15/20/30/40/60/80 mg; 1 tablet bid–tid

Methadone
Methadone 5 mg; 1 tablet q8h #90
Methadone 5/10; 1–5 tablets q8h–q12h; #60–120

Methadone Elixir 5 mg/1 mL; 5 mL (=25 mg) bid–qid
Methadone Elixir 10 mg/5 mL (=2 mg/mL); 5 mL (=10 mg) bid–qid

Ketamine
Dextromethorphan 30/50/75/100 mg capsules

Syrup 5 mg/mL; 1 mL tid; #100 mL
Syrup 10 mg/mL; 1 mL tid; #100 mL

Constipation
Colace 100 mg; 1 tablet tid; #90 (Rely primarily on senokot for opioid-induced constipation)

Relistor <38 kg: 1.5 mg/kg SC every other day PRN; max 1 dose/24 h
Relistor 38–61 kg: 8 mg SC every other day PRN; max 1 dose/24 h
Relistor 62–114 kg: 12 mg SC every other day PRN; max 1 dose/24 h
Relistor 114 kg: 0.15 mg/kg SC every other day PRN; max 1 dose/24 h
Senokot 8.6 mg; 2 tablets qhs; #60
Senokot 8.6 mg; 2–4 tablets bid; max 8 tablets/day; #240

Nausea
Reglan 5 mg; 1 tablet tid; #90
Reglan 10 mg; 1 tablet tid; #90

Suggested Outpatient Medication Prescriptions (Continued)

Stimulants
Provigil (Modafinil) 100/200 mg; 1 tablet qam; max 400 mg/day; #30
Ritalin (Methylphenidate) 10/20 mg; ½–1 tablet at q7am and q11am; #60

TCAs
Amitriptyline (Elavil) 10 mg; 1 tablet qhs–bid; #30–60

Desipramine (Norpramin) 10 mg; 1 tablet qhs–bid; #30–60 (Most Activating)

Nortriptyline (Pamelor) 10 mg; 1 tablet qhs–bid; #30–60
Nortriptyline Oral Solution 10 mg/5 mL; 5 mL qhs–bid; #1 pt

Suggested Compounded Gels
Ketoprofen 10%, Ketamine 10%, Baclofen 2% PLO gel; apply tid; #60 g
Ketoprofen 10% PLO gel; apply tid; #60 g
Ketamine 10%, Gabapentin 6%, Clonidine 0.2% PLO gel; apply tid #60 g

Rectal Fissures, Hemorrhoids
Diltiazem 2%, Lidocaine 5%, apply tid, #30 g
Mouthwash Formula: Tetracycline 62.5 mg/5 mL, Nystatin 60 K
Vaginal Cream: Gabapentin 6% in Acid Mantle Vaginal Cream, insert 1 g
   vaginally bid, #60 g
Vaginal Suppository: Baclofen 20 mg, insert 1 supp vag/rectally bid–qid
   Hoag Eosphagitis Formula: Equal Parts: Maalox Susp, Diphenhydramine
   Liquid 12.5 mg/5 mL, Lidocaine Viscous, Nystatin Ssp (100 M/U/mL),
   swish and swallow 1–2 t Q3–4 hr PRN pain, #240 mL
U/5 mL, Hydrocortisone 2.5 mg/5 mL, Diphenhydramine Liquid
12.5 mg/5 mL × 60 mL, Lidocaine HCL 25 mg/5 mL, Simple Syrup 50 mL,
   rinse mouth with 1 t qid (hold for 2 min) then expectorate, #240 mL

Sleep
Ambien 5/10 mg; 1 tablet qhs; #30
Ambien CR 6.25/12.5 mg; 1 tablet qhs; #30
Lunesta 1/2/3 mg; 1 tablet qhs; #30
Trazodone 50/100 mg; 1–4 tablets qhs; max 400 mg/d; #30–120

---

*See also titration charts, pp. 29–30.

Sample Titration Schedules

Gabapentin
Tablets: 100 mg each

Days	AM	Lunch	QHS
1–3	1	1	1
4–6	1	1	3
7–9	1	3	3
10+	3	3	3

Nortriptyline*
Tablets: 25 mg each

Days	QHS
1–7	1
8–14	2
15–21	3
22–25	4
26–31	5
32–35	6

Amitriptyline*
Tablets: 10 mg each

Days	QHS
1–7	1
8–14	2
15–20	3
21–25	4
26–31	5
32–35	6

*If complete pain relief occurs, halt further increases and continue dose.

Mexilitine
Tablets: 150 mg

Days	AM	Lunch	QHS
1–3	0	0	1
4–6	1	0	1
7–9	1	1	1
10–12	1	1	2
13–16	2	1	2
17+	2	2	2

Sample Titration Schedules (Continued)

Carbamazepine
100 mg

Days	AM	Lunch	QHS
1–3	0	0	1
4–6	1	0	1
7–9	1	1	1
10–12	1	1	2
13–16	2	1	2
17+	2	2	2

Topiramate/Oxcarbazepine
25 mg/150 mg

Days	AM	QHS
1–4	0	1
5–8	1	1
9–12	1	2
13–16	2	2
17–20	2	3
21–24	3	3
25–28	3	4
29+	4	4

Lamotrigine
25 mg

Days	AM	QHS
1–7	0	1
8–14	1	1
15–21	1	2
22–28	2	2
29–34	2	4
35+	4	4

Metabolic Considerations
for Medications

Metabolism
Morphine is hepatically metabolized by glucoronidation; metabolites are excreted renally
M6: causes most common side effects
M3: causes neuroexcitation (myoclonus) and hyperalgesia

Codeine metabolizes to morphine heroin (Di-acetyl-morphine) metabolizes to morphine via deacetylation to 6-mono-acetylmorphine then morphine: Heroin is more water soluble and more potent than morphine

Hydrocodone metabolizes to hydromorphone; therefore, its metabolite has greater activity

Tramadol's M1 metabolite has greater activity than its parent

No active metabolites: Fentanyl; methadone

Enzyme Systems: P2D6
Inhibitors: Codeine, HC, OC, SSRIs
(except superselective SSRIs, such as citalopram and escitalopram, Tramadol, Methadone (although major is 3A4)

Inducers: Carbamazepine

Remember: Tramadol and HC have metabolites with greater analgesia than parent compound

Enzyme Systems: 3A4
Inhibitors: TCAs, morphine, methadone, propoxyphene, erythromycin, benzodiazepines, propanolol, ciprofloxacin, rifampin, INH, cimetidine, grapefruit juice, Fentanyl, warfarin, cyclosporine, theophylline

Inducers: Barbituates, Phenytoin

Metabolic Phases
I: hydrolysis, oxidation, reduction
II: conjugation

What is the difference among MS Contin, OxyContin, and Morphine IR; Morphine CR, and oxycodone IR and CR?

MS Contin = Morphine CR = Morphine Sustained Release = Morphine Controlled Release

Morphine Sulfate IR = Short Acting = Immediate Release

OxyContin = Oxycodone CR = Oxycodone Sustained Release = Oxycodone Controlled Release

Oxycodone IR = Short Acting = Immediate Release

Medication Safety in Renal Failure, Pregnancy, Geriatrics

Renal Failure
Safer in renal failure: Fentanyl, methadone, hydromorphone (some caution)

Pregnancy

Category	Medication
Category A	MVI
Category B	Acetaminophen, caffeine, butorphanol, nalbuphine, fentanyl, hydrocodone, oxycodone, oxymorphone, methadone, mepiridine, morphine, ibuprofen, naprosyn, indomethacin, metoprolol, paroxetine, fluoxetine, prednisone, prednisolone
Category C	Asa, ketorolac, codeine, propoxyphene, gabapentin, lidocaine, mexilitine, nifedipine, propanolol, sumatriptan
Category D	TCA, benzodiazepine, barbiturates, phenytoin, valproate (causes NTDs)
Category X	Ergotamines

Most opioids are Category B.
Avoid: Codeine, propoxyphene, Demerol.
Avoid: Ergots!
Avoid: Antiepileptics (Category D) except Gabapentin (Category C)
Avoid: TCAs (Category D)
Avoid: NSAIDs after 32 weeks*
Avoid: Opioid agonists at high doses near term (13 weeks/term)

Epidural steroids okay in pregnancy
NSAIDs after 32 weeks associated with reversible oligohydramnios.
Diazepam is associated with cleft lip/palate

Lactation
Okay in lactation: Morphine, hydrocodone, hydromorphone, methadone ≤20 mg/day

Safest drugs in lactation: High molecular weight, high ionization, low lipid solubility, and highly protein bound local anesthetics are safe.
Avoid: lithium, cyclosporine, antineoplastic agents, illicit drugs, ergotamines, and bromocriptine (suppresses lactation).

Geriatrics

Decreased renal function, glomerular filtration rate, creatinine clearance, renal blood flow.

Increased plasma drug concentration, terminal half-life.

Decreased Phase I metabolism (hepatic): demethylation, oxidation; decreased liver mass

No change in Phase II metabolism

Decreased albumin levels, increased distribution of meds in plasma, decreased lean body mass, decreased body water, increased fatty tissues.

Increases in lipophilic meds and decreases in hydrophilic meds.

Increased BP (systolic only), pulse pressure.

Decreases in all sensory modalities, except increase in nociception.

Interventional Pharmacology

Local Anesthetic Agent	Concentrations (%)	Onset/ Duration	Recommended Max Single Dose w/o Epi	Toxic Dose
Lidocaine	0.5, 1, 1.5, 2.5	Fast/ 30–60 min	300 mg	4.5 mg/kg
Bupivacaine	0.25, 0.5, 0.75	Slow/ 120–240 min	175 mg	2 mg/kg

Source: Chart adapted from Botelho RJ, Sitzman BT. Pharmacology for the interventional pain physician. *Essentials of Pain Medicine* (Chap. 19, 3rd edition).

Local Anesthetic Adverse Reactions

CNS Toxicity: Proportional to potency of LA and serum blood level. Initial symptoms are usually excitatory (blockade of central inhibitory pathways).

In order of appearance:
1. Numbness of tongue or foreign taste, 2. Lightheadedness, 3. Auditory disturbances, 4. Muscular twitching, 5. Unconsciousness, 6. Convulsions, 7. Coma, 8. Respiratory arrest, 9. Cardiovascular depression

Cardiovascular Toxicity: Most LA will not produce CV toxicity until blood levels are 2× that to produce seizures. LA bind to and inhibit cardiac Na channels (Bupivacaine binds more avidly and with longer duration)

Neuronal Toxicity: 1. Preservative related, 2. LA concentration related—5% lidocaine Vasoconstrictor (when Epi is used): Tachycardia, HTN, HA, Apprehension

Allergic Reactions: Most common with esters > amides: 1. Vasomotor (warmth, flush), 2. Cutaneous (hives, urticaria), 3. Bronchospasm (wheezing), 4. Cardiovascular (hypotension), 5. Vasovagal (bradycardia, hypotension, nausea), 6. Anaphylaxis (angioedema, urticaria, bronchospasm, hypotension)

Absorption Is Dependent on the Vascularity of the Injection Site:
Subcutaneous > intercostal > caudal > epidural >
peripheral nerve > intrathecal

Interventional Pharmacology (Continued)

Glucocorticoid Agent	Half-Life (h)	Anti-inflammatory Potency	Salt-Retaining Potency	Particulate Size (Aggregation)
Hydrocortisone	8–12	1	1	
Triamcinolone	12–36	5	0	<RBC size to 13× (dense)
Methylprednisolone	12–36	5	0.5	<RBC size (dense)
Dexamethasone	36–72	25	0	<RBC size (none)
Betamethasone	36–72	25	0	Varied (dense)

Adverse Reactions Associated With Corticosteroids

Fluid retention, HTN, hyperglycemia, generalized erythema/facial flushing, menstrual irregularities, gastritis/PUD, hypothalamic–pituitary–adrenal axis suppression, Cushing Syndrome, bone demineralization, steroid myopathy, allergic reaction

Adverse Reactions to Contrast Agents

Chemotoxic: Thyrotoxicosis, nephrotoxicity
Hyperosmolalic: Erythrocyte damage, endothelial damage and thrombosis, vasodilation, hypervolemia, cardiac depression
Allergic: Vasomotor, cutaneous, bronchospasm, cardiovascular, vasovagal, anaphylaxis.

Treatment: Diphenhydramine, 25 mg IV

Interventional Pharmacology (Continued)

■ 2010 ASRA RECOMMENDATIONS FOR ANTICOAGULATION IN PAIN MEDICINE PROCEDURES

Medication	Recommendation
Unfractionated Heparin SQ	Preferable to perform injection prior to heparin SQ. No increased risk of neuraxial block with heparin SQ
NSAID	Grade 1A: No additional risk of spinal epidural hematoma
ASA	Grade 1A: No additional risk of spinal epidural hematoma
Ticlopidine	Discontinue 14 days prior to neuraxial block
Clopidogrel	Discontinue 7 days prior to neuraxial block
GP IIb/IIIa	Use is contraindicated within 4-week period of surgery. If neuraxial technique must be performed, monitor neurologic status.
Thrombin Inhibitors	Grade 2C: recommend against neuraxial blocks
Fondaparinux	Unknown due to limited literature, recommend single needle, atraumatic placement, and avoiding catheters.
Rivaroxaben	Unknown due to limited literature, recommend caution due to prolonged half-life
Herbal Medication	Grade 1C: No additional risk

(Continued)

Medication	Prior to Needle Placement	After Needle Placement	Catheter Discontinuation
Unfractionated Heparin IV	No formal recommendation. IV heparin has half life of 60–90 minutes. Can reverse 100U heparin with 1 mg of protamine	May begin heparin IV 1 hr after needle placed	Should discontinue heparin IV 2–4 hr prior to discontinuing neuraxial catheter. Monitor sensory and motor function 12 hr after discontinuing catheter
Low-Molecular Weight Heparin (LMWH)	Grade 1C: Discontinue prophylactic dose 10–12 hr prior to needle placed Grade 1C: Discontinue treatment dose 24 hr prior to needle placed	Grade 2C: Start LMWH 24 hr after needle placement	Discontinue catheter 10–12 hr after LMWH stopped, may restart LMWH 2 hr after catheter removed
Warfarin	Grade 1B: Discontinue warfarin 4–5 days prior to neuraxial block. INR must be normalized	No formal recommendation	Grade 2C: Discontinue neuraxial catheters when INR <1.5 and monitor neurological function at least 24 hr after catheter discontinued

▉ EMERGENCY PHARMACOLOGY

Hypotension, HR <60
▉ Ephedrine 5 mg
▉ Intravenous fluids

Hypotension, HR >60
▉ Neosynepherine 100 mcg IVP (dilute 1:100)
▉ Intravenous fluids

Hypertension
▉ Labetolol 5 mg IVP
▉ Metoprolol 5 mg IVP
▉ Esmolol 10 mg IVP
▉ Hydralazine

Bradycardia
▉ Glycopyrolate 0.2 mg IVP
▉ Ephedrine 5 mg IVP (dilute 1:10)

Tachycardia, SBP >110
▉ Esmolol 10 mg IVP

Tachycardia With Hypotension
▉ Neosynephrine 100 mcg

Seizures
▉ Versed 2 mg IVP
▉ Propofol 50 mg IVP
▉ Oxygen
▉ ABCs

Local Anesthetic Toxicity
▉ 1.5 mL/kg 20% lipid emulsion bolus
▉ 0.25 mL/kg/min of infusion, continued for at least 10 min after circulatory stability attained
▉ If circulatory stability not attained, consider rebolus and increasing infusion to 0.5 mL/kg/min
▉ 10 mL/kg lipid emulsion for 30 min is recommended as the upper limit for initial dosing

▓ INTRATHECAL PUMP

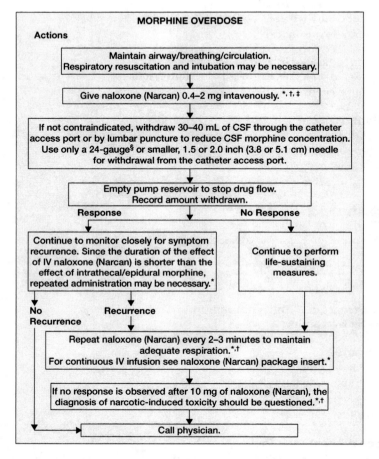

Figure 1.1 Morphine intrathecal/epidural overdose emergency procedures.

* Infumorph (preservative-free morphine sulfate sterile solution) manufacturer's package insert (Wyeth-Ayerst).

† Narcan (naloxone hydrochloride) manufacturer's package insert (DuPont).

‡ Refer to the drug manufacturer's package insert for a complete list of indications, contraindications, warnings, precautions, adverse events, and dosage and dosage and administration information.

§ Use a 25-gauge needle for withdrawal from a SynchroMed II or IsoMed catheter access port.

Adapted from Metronic: Indications, drug stability, and emergency procedures. SynchroMed and IsoMed implantable infusion systems.

▓ INTRATHECAL PUMP (*Continued*)

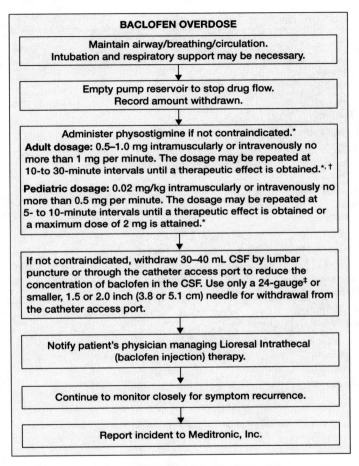

BACLOFEN OVERDOSE

Maintain airway/breathing/circulation.
Intubation and respiratory support may be necessary.

↓

Empty pump reservoir to stop drug flow.
Record amount withdrawn.

↓

Administer physostigmine if not contraindicated.*
Adult dosage: 0.5–1.0 mg intramuscularly or intravenously no
more than 1 mg per minute. The dosage may be repeated at
10-to 30-minute intervals until a therapeutic effect is obtained.*, †

Pediatric dosage: 0.02 mg/kg intramuscularly or intravenously no
more than 0.5 mg per minute. The dosage may be repeated at
5- to 10-minute intervals until a therapeutic effect is obtained or
a maximum dose of 2 mg is attained.*

↓

If not contraindicated, withdraw 30–40 mL CSF by lumbar
puncture or through the catheter access port to reduce the
concentration of baclofen in the CSF. Use only a 24-gauge‡ or
smaller, 1.5 or 2.0 inch (3.8 or 5.1 cm) needle for withdrawal from
the catheter access port.

↓

Notify patient's physician managing Lioresal Intrathecal
(baclofen injection) therapy.

↓

Continue to monitor closely for symptom recurrence.

↓

Report incident to Meditronic, Inc.

**Figure 1.2 Lioresal Intrathecal (baclofen injection) overdose emergncy
procedures.**

* Refer to the drug manufacturer's package insert for a complete list of indications,
contraindications, warnings, precautions, adverse events, and dosage and
administration information.
† Müller-Schwefe G, Penn RD. Physostigmine in the treatment of intrathecal baclofen
overdose: Report of three cases. *J Neurosurg.* August 1989;71:279–275.
‡ Use a 25-gauge needle for withdrawal from a SynchroMed or SynchroMed
EL catheter access port. Use a 24- or 25-gauge needle for withdrawal from a
SynchroMed II or IsoMed catheter access port.

Adapted from Metronic: Indications, drug stability, and emergency procedures.
SynchroMed and IsoMed implantable infusion systems.

▧ INTRATHECAL PUMP (*Continued*)

DRUG STABILITY

	SynchroMed II	SynchroMed and SynchroMed EL	IsoMed
Cisplatin 1 mg/mL	—	7 days	—
Clindamycin 70 mg/mL	—	28 days	—
Doxorubicin 5 mg/mL	—	14 days	—
Floxuridine 20 mg/mL	56 days	28 days	27 days
Lioresal intrathecal 0.5 mg/mL, 2 mg/mL	180 days	90 days	—
Methotrexate 5 mg/mL	56 days	28 days	—
Morphine Sulfate 25 mg/mL	180 days	90 days	90 days
Ziconotide	Initial fill	Refill	
25 mcg/mL undiluted	14 days	60 days	
100 mcg/mL undiluted		60 days	
100 mcg/mL diluted		40 days	

■ SYSTEMIC EFFECTS OF LOCAL ANESTHETICS

Plasma Lidocaine Concentration (mcg/mL)	Effect
1–5	Analgesia
5–10	Lightheadedness, tinnitus, numbness of the tongue
10–15	Seizures, unconsciousness
15–25	Coma, respiratory arrest
>25	Cardiovascular depression

Agent	Relative Potency for CNS Toxicity	CVS:CNS
Bupivacaine	4	2.0
Levobupivacaine	2.9	2.0
Chloroprocaine	0.3	3.7
Etidocaine	2.0	4.4
Lidocaine	1.0	7.1
Mepivacaine	1.4	7.1
Prilocaine	1.2	3.1
Procaine	0.3	3.7
Ropivacaine	2.9	2.2
Tetracaine	2.0	—

LIDOCAINE 1% MAX DOSING CHART: ADULTS

Weight (kg)	Weight (lb)	Max Dose (mg)	Max Dose (mL)
30	66	135	13.5
40	88	180	18.0
50	110	225	22.5
60	132	275	27.5
>66	>145	300	30

Maximum dose: 4.5 mg/kg or 300 mg total
Lidocaine 1% = 10 mg/mL

BUPIVICAINE 0.25% MAX DOSING CHART: ADULTS

Weight (kg)	Weight (lbs)	Max Dose (mg)	Max Dose (mL)
30	66	60	24
40	88	80	32
50	110	100	40
60	132	120	48
70	154	140	56
80	176	160	64
>87	>190	175	70

Maximum dose: 2 mg/kg or 175 mg/dose
Bupivicaine 0.25% = 2.5 mg/mL

Traditional Neurolytic Spinal Blocks

	Alcohol	Phenol
Physical properties	Low water solubility	Absorbs water on air exposure
Stability at room temperature	Unstable	Stable
Concentration	100%	4–7%
Diluent	None	Glycerin
Relative to CSF	Hypobaric	Hyperbaric
Patient position	Lateral	Lateral
Added tilt	Semi prone	Semi supine
Painful side	Uppermost	Most dependent
Injection sensations	Immediate burning pain	Painless, warm feeling
Onset of neurolysis	Immediate	Delayed 15 min
CSF uptake	30 min	15 min
Full effect	3–5 d	1 d
Mechanism	Extract lipids; precipitates proteins	Coagulates proteins

Source: Chart adapted from Hurley, RW, Ellis N, Adams, MCB. Central and Peripheral Neurolysis. *Essesntials of Pain Medicine and Regional Anesthesia* (Chap. 72, 3rd edition).

Botox Injections for Migraine

Mechanism of Action

Inhibits the release of neurotransmitters such as acetylcholine by entering the presynaptic neurons and cleaving proteins responsible for docking and fusion of the synaptic vesicles to the presynaptic membrane. Type B acts on the outside of the synaptic vesicle, cleaving the vesicle-associated membrane protein (VAMP, synaptobrevin), whereas type A acts on the inner surface of the postsynaptic membrane (synaptosomal-associated protein of 25sd, SNAP-25). In addition to inhibiting acetylcholine release, botulinum toxin also appears to inhibit other neurotransmitters such as noradrenaline, dopamine, gamma-aminobutyrate, Glycine, peptide methionine-enkephalin, as well as the pain nociceptor substance P. In the muscle, botulinum toxin inhibits the release of acetylcholine at the neuromuscular junction of the muscle fibers and at the muscle spindles. In the periphery, botulinum toxin may reduce the release of pain nociceptors.

Allergan for Practioners	1-800-433-8871
Botox Information Line	1-800-44-Botox www.allergan.com www.botox.com
Solstice Neurosciences	1-888-461-2255
Myobloc Information	www.solsticeneuro.com

Frequency of Injection: The duration of benefit lasts 3–6 months.

Source: Odderson R. *Botulinum Toxin Injection Guide*. Demos 2008.

Botox Injections for Migraine (Continued)

MIGRAINE DOSING RANGES

	Botox	Myobloc	Injection Sites per Muscle
Procerus	2.5–5.0/site	50–100	1
Corrugator, medial	2.5–4.0/site	Limited data	1
Frontalis	2.5/site (4–6/side)	500–750	8–12
Temporalis, each muscle	2.5–5/site (4/side)	Limited data	4
Occipitalis	5–10/side	Limited data	1
Splenius capitis	5–15/side	Limited data	1–2
Masseter	5–15/side	Limited data	1–2
L. Scapulae	10–25/side	Limited data	
Trapezius	5–15/side	625–1000/side	1–3
Semispinalis	5–10/side	Limited data	1
SCM	10–20/side	Limited data	2
Total dose	100–200	2500–5000	
Dilution	100 U/2–4 mL, dispensed in 1 mL syringes		
Needle	30 G, 0.5 in.		

Facial injections are done bilaterally to avoid asymmetric expressions. Avoid injections into the brow areas; inject approximately 2 cm above the brows. Follow-the-pain: This approach for injections allows a more individualized approach depending on the patient's localization of pain and tender/trigger points.

Botox Injection Sites for Migraine

Muscles possibly involved	Migraine 1/3

Muscles possibly involved

Procerus
Corrugator
Frontalis
Temporalis
Occipitalis
Splenius capitis
Masseter
Levator scapulae
Trapezius
Sternocleidomastoid
Cervical paraspinal muscles

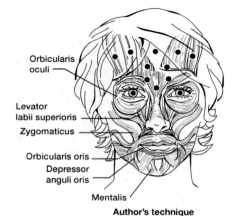

Orbicularis oculi

Levator labii superioris

Zygomaticus

Orbicularis oris

Depressor anguli oris

Mentalis

Author's technique

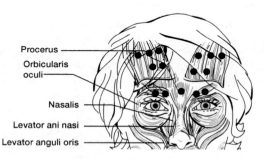

Procerus

Orbicularis oculi

Nasalis

Levator ani nasi

Levator anguli oris

Blumenfeld technique

Muscles possibly involved

Procerus
Corrugator
Frontalis
Temporalis
Occipitalis
Masseter
Levator scapulae
Sternocleidomastoid
Splenius capitis
Trapezius
Cervical paraspinal muscles

Migraine 2/3

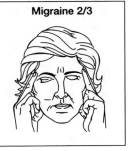

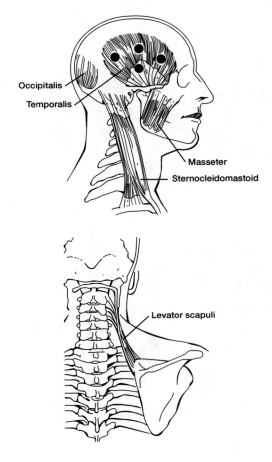

Occipitalis

Temporalis

Masseter

Sternocleidomastoid

Levator scapuli

Muscles possibly involved	Migraine 3/3
Procerus	
Corrugator	
Frontalis	
Temporalis	
Occipitalis	
Masseter	
Sternocleidomastoid	
Levator scapulae	
Splenius capitis	
Trapezius	
Cervical paraspinal muscles	

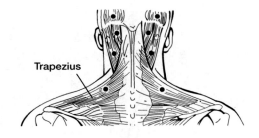

Trapezius

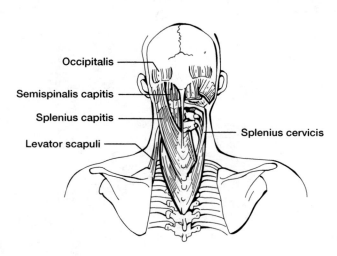

Occipitalis

Semispinalis capitis

Splenius capitis

Levator scapuli

Splenius cervicis

Note
5 mL = 1 teaspoon (t); 15 mL = 1 tablespoon (T)

How to Present Pain

Location

Radiation

Intermittent Versus Continuous

Frequency; Duration

Onset: Sudden or Insidious

Description (Nociceptive or Neuropathic or Mixed)

Intensity: Visual Analog Scale Scores

Exacerbating Factors; Alleviating Factors

Associated Symptoms

Numbness/Tingling/Weakness?

Bowel or Bladder Changes?

Headaches

Presentation	Treatment
Tension/cervicogenic	
▓ Nonvascular ▓ Women > men ▓ Not familial ▓ Usually bilateral ▓ Onset 4–8 am/pm ▓ Secondary to stress and/or c-spine pathology ▓ Frequency: 15 or more days/month over a minimum of 3 months	▓ Abortive: acetaminophen, NSAIDs, caffeine ▓ Prophylactic: antidepressants, TCA, anticonvulsants, beta blockers
Migraine	
▓ Unilateral ▓ Women > men ▓ Familial presents before age 30 ▓ Lasts 4–24 hrs ▓ Vascular, throbbing, pounding, retro-orbital, ± n/v, phono/photophobia, ± aura (classic vs common) ▓ Associated with anxiety, bipolar D/O (10%) ▓ Triggers: menstruation, OCPs, tyrosine, alcohol, physical activity	▓ Abortive: Isometheptene Mucate (Midrin = sympathomimetic), triptans, ergots, oxygen, IV lidocaine, IV droperidol, naproxen ▓ Prophylactic: beta-blockers, CCBs, antidepressants, clonidine, gabapentin, antiepileptics, methysergide (in refractory cases; associated with cardiac fibrosis)
Basilar migraine	
▓ Women > men ▓ Visual disturbances common, may evolve into blindness ▓ Differs from migraine in character and severity of neurologic deficit, ± irritability, frank psychosis, transient tetraplegia, stupor, syncope, coma ▓ May last hours	▓ See treatment for migraine

Headaches *(Continued)*

Presentation	Treatment
Cluster	
▓ Men > women ▓ Occurs within 90 min of falling asleep ▓ Not familial ▓ Occurs 2–3 times a day ▓ Each attack lasts about 1 hr ▓ Temporal, retro-orbital area ▓ Clusters for about 10 wks, remission about 6–8 mo ▓ Symptoms develops in 30s ▓ Increased in spring and fall	▓ Oxygen, methysergide, oral corticosteroids, lithium, indomethacin, sphenopalatine block, RF Gasserian ganglion
Paroxysmal hemicranias	
▓ Similar to cluster type, benign ▓ Poor response to anticluster meds except indomethacin, which is treatment of choice and whose response determines the diagnosis ▓ Severe, throbbing, orbital or supraorbital, or temporal, ± conjunctival injection, lacrimation, nasal congestion, rhinorrhea, ptosis, eyelid edema, usually >8 attacks/24 hr	▓ Indomethacin
Occipital neuralgia	
▓ Suboccipital, aching, throbbing, radiates to posterolateral scalp, usually worse toward end of day, ± scalp hyperesthesia	▓ GON block
Sinusitis	
▓ Maxillary tenderness ▓ CT: air fluid level or >8 mm thickening	▓ Abx 14–21 days; nasal saline sprays
Posttraumatic HA (postconcussive)	
▓ CT: R/O SDH, NPH	▓ Depakote (check CBC, LFTs), Gabapentin

Headaches (Continued)

Presentation	Treatment
Trigeminal neuralgia	
▓ V2 or V3 distribution, secondary to aberrant blood vessels irritating or pressing on the trigeminal nerve ▓ Associated with MS (rule out MS if age <30), acoustic neuromas, bony abnormalities, aneurysms ▓ Paroxysmal, electric pain lasts seconds to minutes, + trigger points around upper lip, nose ▓ Tic Douloureux: painful facial muscle spasms on ipsilateral side (patient to avoid talking, eating, touching face), patient grimaces to immobilize any trigger zones	▓ Gabapentin, carbamazepine (watch for aplastic anemia), baclofen, phenytoin
TMJ	
▓ Triggered by movement of jaw, yawning, eating, chewing ▓ Dull, continuous, poorly localized pain, achy, gnawing, ± cramping, jaw locking ▓ Usually self-limited, associated with TMJ-disc prolapses in an anterior or anteromedial direction, ear fullness, periauricular pain ▓ PE: auscultate for clicks. Mandible may deviate toward affected side until disc prolapses back into place. Jaw opening is diminished usually <40 mm. Hard clicking late in jaw opening (at >25 mm) = pathologic joint changes	▓ Intracapsular pathology: dental splints at night + stretching + corticosteroid injection ▓ Extracapsular (associated with masseter muscle pathology): TPI ▓ Can also try hypnosis
Giant cell arteritis, temporal arteritis, cranial arteritis, Horton's syndrome	
▓ Jaw claudication, elevated ESR, granulomatous inflammation to medium-sized blood vessels, 90% + HA, may cause blindness, median age = 70, head/scalp soreness, associated with polymyalgia rheumatica (PMR)	▓ Corticosteroids

Headaches (Continued)

Presentation	Treatment
Herpes zoster (V1 distribution)	
▓ Severe HA, weak eyelid muscles	▓ Acyclovir, famciclovir,
▓ Argyll–Robinson pupil: pupil accommodates but does not react to light	valacyclovir
	▓ Analgesics
▓ ± Bell's Palsy	
▓ Lesions on face, cornea, mouth, tongue	
▓ May cause vertigo, hearing deficits, vesicular rash around external ear canal	
Pseudomotor cerebri	
▓ Benign intracranial HTN, CSF pressure >300 mm Hg	▓ Acetazolamide
	▓ Lumbar puncture
▓ + papilledema	
▓ More common in women > men, age 30–40 yrs	

Cranial Nerve Notes and Pain Boards Association

CN No.	Sensory (S), Motor (M), Both (B)	Name	Skull Exit	Notes
I	S	Olfactory	Cribriform plate	▪ (Most common injury CN in TBI)
II	S	Optic	Optic canal w/ophthalmic artery	▪ Corneal anesthesia
III	M	Oculomotor	Superior orbital fissure	▪ Innervates inferior oblique, medial, and inferior rectus
IV	M	Trochlear	Superior orbital fissure	▪ Only CN to exit brainstem from the dorsal surface ▪ Innervates superior oblique muscle of the orbit
V1	S	Ophthalmic	Superior orbital fissure	▪ Frontal N (supraorbital and supratrochlear branches) innervates upper eyelid, forehead, and scalp ▪ Nasocilliary (infratrochlear and external nasal branches) innervates apex/ala of nose and anterior nasal cavity ▪ Lacrimal N innervates gland, outer canthus of eye

Cranial Nerve Notes and Pain Boards Association (Continued)

CN No.	Sensory (S), Motor (M), Both (B)	Name	Course	Notes
V2	S	Maxillary	Exits foramen rotundum to pterygopalatine fossa, emerges on face via infra-orbital foramen	▪ Middle meningeal N to dura of middle cranial fossa ▪ Zygomatic N to zygomatic region, mucosa of maxillary sinus, upper gums/molars, cheek mucous membranes ▪ Ant-Sup alveolar and middle Sup N to incisors, canines, Ant wall of the maxillary antrum, floor of nasal cavity, premolars ▪ Inferior palpebral N to conjunctiva, skin of low eyelid ▪ External nasal N to side of nose ▪ Sup labial N to upper lip, oral mucosa
V3	B	Mandibular	Foramen ovale	▪ Lingual N innervates mandible, dorsal-anterior surface of tongue ▪ Auriculotemporal N innervates teeth of lower jaw, external auditory meatus, temporal region, anterior ear, TMJ, skin over lower third of face
VI	M	Abducens	Superior orbital fissure	▪ Innervates lateral rectus of orbit
VII	B	Facial	Internal auditory meatus	▪ Innervates orbicularis oris, buccinator

Cranial Nerve Notes and Pain Boards Association (*Continued*)

CN No.	Sensory (S), Motor (M), Both (B)	Name	Course	Notes
VIII	S	Vestibulo-cochlear	Internal auditory meatus	▪ Hearing and vestibular system
IX	B	Glosso-pharyngeal	Jugular foramen	▪ Innervates: palatine tonsils, posterior third of tongue, hypopharynx and pharynx
X	M	Vagus	Jugular foramen	▪ Innervates base of tongue, epiglottis, larynx, trachea ▪ Superior laryngeal N blocked as it passes below the greater cornu of the hyoid bone. Branches: (1) Internal laryngeal N (supplies sensation from the epiglottis to the VC), (2) external laryngeal N (innervates cricothyroid muscle, tenses VC) ▪ Recurrent laryngeal N (RLN): supplies sensation below the VC and inner-vates all laryngeal muscles except cricothyroid. Runs between trachea and esophagus, may be inadvertently blocked following stellate ganglion block. RLN enters the larynx posterior to the cricothyroid articulation and can be blocked by a transtracheal approach through the cricothyroid membrane

Cranial Nerve Notes and Pain Boards Association (Continued)

CN No.	Sensory (S), Motor (M), Both (B)	Name	Course	Notes
XI	M	Accessory	Jugular foramen	▦ Innervates trapezius
XII	M	Hypoglossal	Hypoglossal canal	▦ To hypopharynx, sensation to posterior tongue, motor to tongue

Facial Pain Neuralgias

Type	Presentation	Treatment
Trigeminal neuralgia	▦ V2 or V3 distribution, secondary to aberrant blood vessels irritating or pressing on the trigeminal nerve ▦ Associated with MS, (rule out MS if < age 30), acoustic neuromas, bony abnormalities, aneurysms ▦ Paroxysmal, electric pain, lasts seconds to minutes, + trigger points around upper lip, nose ▦ Tic Doloreaux: painful facial muscle spasms on ipsilateral side (pt avoid talking, eating, touching face), patient grimaces to immobilize any trigger zones	▦ Gabapentin, carbamazepine (watch for aplastic anemia), baclofen, phenytoin
Geniculate neuralgia	▦ Nervus intermedius branch of CN VII ▦ Deep ear pain, may cause vertigo, tinnitus ▦ Ramsay–Hunt syndrome: H. Zoster of the geniculate ganglion ▦ Triggers: talking, swallowing, ear contact	▦ Gabapentin, carbamazepine (watch for aplastic anemia), baclofen, phenytoin
Glossopharyngeal neuralgia	▦ Paroxysmal lancinating pain, unilateral, brief but multiple attacks, may be secondary to tumor infiltration, may cause syncope, arrhythmias ▦ Triggers: talking, chewing, odynophagia	▦ Gabapentin, carbamazepine (watch for aplastic anemia), baclofen, phenytoin

Facial Pain Neuralgias (Continued)

Type	Presentation	Treatment
Superior laryngeal neuralgia	▨ Associated with hiccups, cough ▨ Pain: larynx, throat, angle of jaw ▨ Triggers: coughing, swallowing, yawning, talking	▨ Carbamazepine ▨ Superior laryngeal nerve block
Occipital neuralgia	▨ GON (dorsal rami of C2, C3) ± LON (C2–C4 via cervical plexus): unilateral local tenderness, suboccipital, radiates to posterolateral scalp, ± scalp hyperesthesia ▨ Pain usually worse at end of the day ▨ Triggers: head movement	▨ GON block
Deafferentation pain	▨ Etiology from cordotomy or neurolysis (RFA, phenol, alcohol) for neuropathic pain syndromes (PHN, thalamic pain, SCI, CRPS, phantom pain)	▨ Carbamazepine, anticonvulsants, TCA, clonazepam, topiramate

Pelvic Pain Neuralgias

Type	Notes
Iliohypogastric nerve L1–L2	Suprapubic sensation
Ilioinguinal nerve L1–L2	Sensation over inguinal ligament, base of penis, base of scrotum or labia
Genitofemoral nerve L1–L2	Lateral scrotum, vulva, cremaster muscle
Pudendal nerve S2–S4	Branches include posterior scrotal/labial, dorsal, inferior rectal and perineal nerves (last two innervate anus and anal sphincter)

Gynecologic Conditions That May Cause or Exacerbate Chronic Pelvic Pain by Level of Evidence

Level A: Good and consistent scientific evidence of causal relationship to chronic pelvic pain

- Endometriosis
- Gynecologic malignancies
- Ovarian retention syndrome
- Ovarian remnant syndrome
- Pelvic congestion syndrome
- Pelvic inflammatory disease
- Tuberculous salpingitis

Level B: Limited or inconsistent scientific evidence of causal relationship to chronic pelvic pain

- Adhesions
- Benign cystic mesothelioma
- Leiomyomata
- Postoperative peritoneal cysts

Level C: Casual relationship to chronic pelvic pain based on expert opinions

- Adenomyosis
- Atypical dysmenorrhea or ovulatory pain
- Adnexal cysts
- Cervical stenosis
- Chronic ectopic pregnancy
- Chronic endometritis
- Endometrial or cervical polyps
- Endosalpingiosis
- Intrauterine contraceptive device
- Ovarian ovulatory pain
- Residual accessory ovary
- Symptomatic pelvic relaxation

Nongynecologic Conditions That May Cause or Exacerbate Chronic Pelvic Pain by Level of Evidence

Level of Evidence	Urologic	Gastrointestinal	Musculoskeletal	Other
Level A	Bladder malignancy Interstitial cystitis Radiation cystitis Urethral syndrome	Colon malignancy Constipation Inflammatory bowel disease Irritable bowel syndrome	Abdominal wall myofascial pain Chronic coccygeal or back pain Faulty or poor posture Fibromyalgia Neuralgia of iliohypogastric, ilioinguinal, and/or genitofemoral nerves Pelvic floor myalgias Peripartum pelvic pain syndrome	Abdominal cutaneous nerve entrapment in surgical scar Depression Somatization disorder
Level B	Detrusor dyssynergia Urethral diverticulum		Herniated nucleus propulsus Low back pain Neoplasia of spinal cord or sacral nerve	Celiac disease Neurologic dysfunction Porphyria Shingles Sleep disturbances
Level C	Chronic UTI Recurrent, acute cystitis Recurrent, acute urethritis Stone/urolithiasis Urethral caruncle	Colitis Chronic intermittent bowel obstruction Diverticular disease	Compression of lumbar vertebrae Degenerative joint disease Hernias Muscular strains and sprains Rectus tendon strain Spondylosis	Abdominal epilepsy Abdominal migraine Bipolar personality disorders Familial Mediterranean fever

Source: ACOG Practice Bulletin No. 51. Chronic pelvic pain. Obstet Gynecol. 2004 Mar;103(3):589–605.

Radiology Pearls

MRI: Aligns H+ ions with a + or − spin.

A second electric field causes a charged state. When relaxation occurs, each charged ion emits energy detectable by a radiofrequency receiver.

Each tissue has characteristic relaxation times:
T1: CSF Black, better detail; T2: CSF White

Wavelength is determined by the Larmor equation: Magnetic field strength × gyromagnetic constant

When to use gadolinium (CONTRAST):

1. Postsurgery
2. Infection
3. Tumor

Gadolinium has no iodine and is safe, in general, in renal insufficiency. (However, there are a handful of cases of nephrogenic fibrosing dermapathy.)

MRI Disadvantages: Detects pathology in 20% of asymptomatic individuals; poor facet visualization; poor visualization of neural foraminal narrowing secondary to osteophytes.

MRI Best for: UE/LE Joint disease, LBP, HNP, spinal stenosis, posttrauma, evaluation of vertebral alignment, cervical-thoracic junction, spinal infection, mass lesions.

CT Best for: bone, joints, foraminal bony stenosis.

Modic Changes:

1. Increased signal on T2: vascularized marrow
2. Increased signal on T1: possible Iso- or increased signal on T2: Fatty infiltration of the marrow
3. Decreased signal on T1 and T2: sclerosis

Disc Pathology Pearls

Disc Pathology	Description	Schematic
Bulge	▓ Lax annulus fibrosis (AF) ▓ Presence of outer annulus beyond plane of disc space	
Protrusion	▓ Torn AF (partially intact) ▓ Herniated disc in which the greatest plane, in any direction, between the edges of the disc material beyond the disc space is less than the distance between the edges of the base, when measured in the same plane	
Extrusion	▓ Nucleus pulposus (NP) has ruptured through AF (torn) and bulges into spinal canal or intervertebral foramen ▓ A herniated disc in which, in at least one plane, any one distance between the edges of the disc material beyond the disc space is greater than the distance between the edges of the base in the same plane	
Sequestration	▓ Nucleus pulposus (NP) has ruptured through AF (torn) and bulges into spinal canal or intervertebral foramen ▓ An extruded disc in which a portion of the disc tissue is displaced beyond the outer annulus and maintains no connection by disc tissue with the disc of origin	

IDET Criteria

Success rate 23%–60%: Young patient; preservation of disc height; lumbar discogenic pain; no facet disease/symptoms; no radicular disease/symptoms; concordant positive discography; no prior disc surgery.

Spinal Pain Differential

Axial Spine Pain

- Vertebral body fractures; compression fractures
- Interspinous ligament; ligamentous strain/injury
- Acute muscle strain/injury
- Myofascial pain (regional)
- Facet arthropathy; degenerative joint disease
- Spondylolisthesis (check flex/ext for instability)
- Discogenic disease; annular tear
- Spinal stenosis (can be radicular also)
- Cancer; metastases (worse at PM; constitutional symptoms)
- Scoliosis; pelvic obliquity
- Fibromyalgia (diffuse body involvement)
- Referred pain (renal, pancreas)
- Sacroiliac joint pain
- Hip arthritis (usually also with groin pain)
- Ischial bursitis; greater trocanteric bursitis
- Post-laminectomy pain; hardware-associated pain
- Inflammatory arthropathy
- Infection

Radicular Pain

- Radiculopathy secondary to herniated disc (HNP)
- Radiculopathy secondary to facet arthropathy
- Spinal stenosis (neurogenic claudication)
- Piriformis Syndrome; sciatica
- Lumbosacral plexopathy

Description	Stages	Treatment
Type I (RSD) ▪ A prolonged sympathetic response to an injury ▪ May involve "opening of the gate": damage to A-Beta fibers: allowing for pain transmission	1. Acute or hyperemic stage: Increased blood flow, increased temperature, + erythema. Pain: burning, neuralgic, + allodynia, ± hyper/hypoesthesia 2. Dystrophic stage: Pain: burning, throbbing, widespread and spontaneous, + joint stiffness, decreased blood flow, limb is cool, edematous and mottled, coarse hair, cracked nails with ridges, early osteoporosis, muscle atrophy. Bone scan: increased Static Phase 3. Atrophic stage: Irreversible! marked edema, glossy skin, marked atrophy, osteoporosis, ± spontaneous fractures, large decrease in blood flow, cyanotic appearing, trophic changes, 3+ sudomotor dysfunction. Bone scan: decreased in all phases except the static phase	▪ Stellate ▪ LSB ▪ IV bretylium regional block (causes release of NER and prevents further release: 5–10 mg/kg IV. Side effects: HTN followed by hypotension and ventricular ectopy) ▪ Oral corticosteroids ▪ Gabapentin and other neuropathic medications including TCA, SNRI, and propanolol ▪ Physical therapy: Tactile desensitization, AROM
Type II (causalgia) ▪ 1 mo post-injury onset ▪ Sustained, constant, burning pain, progressing from distal to central, + hyperesthesia, with vaso-sudomotor changes, hair loss, nail changes, atrophy, decalcification, glossy thin skin		

Treatment Considerations for Common Pain Presentations

Presentation	Treatment Considerations
Radiculopathy	▪ Activity modification ▪ Home exercise program—Core strengthening, McKenzie program ▪ Modalities (heat, ice, TENS) ▪ Acupuncture ▪ OMT/manual therapy ▪ Short-term soft lumbar support ▪ Physical therapy, aquatherapy ▪ Oral analgesics (NSAIDs, acetaminophen) ▪ Neuropathic analgesics ▪ Antispasmodics ▪ Opioid analgesics ▪ Interlaminar epidural steroid injections ▪ Transforaminal epidural steroid injections ▪ Caudal epidural steroid injections ▪ Spinal cord stimulation
Sacroiliac	▪ Activity modification ▪ Home exercise program ▪ Modalities (heat, ice, TENS) ▪ Acupuncture ▪ OMT/manual therapy ▪ SIJ bracing ▪ Physical therapy, aquatherapy ▪ Oral analgesics (NSAIDS, acetaminophen) ▪ Opioid analgesics ▪ SI Joint steroid injection ▪ Strip Lesioning ▪ Lateral branch denervation

Treatment Considerations for Common Pain Presentations (Continued)

Presentation	Treatment Considerations
Knee	▓ Activity modification ▓ Weight loss ▓ Supplements (glucosamine/chondroitin) ▓ Durable medical equipment/offloading (walker/cane) ▓ Home exercise program—partial arc quadriceps strengthening ▓ Modalities (heat, ice, iontophoresis) ▓ Acupuncture ▓ Bracing (neoprene vs offloader vs other) ▓ Medial vs lateral heel wedge for valgus vs varus deformity ▓ Physical therapy, aquatherapy ▓ Oral analgesics (NSAIDs, acetaminophen) ▓ Topical analgesics (capsaicin) ▓ Opioid analgesics ▓ Knee intra-articular steroid injection ▓ Hyaluronic Acid Series Injection ▓ RF/Pulsed RF of Intra-articular surfaces ▓ Nerve block—saphenous
Intra-articular hip	▓ Activity modification ▓ Weight loss ▓ Home exercise program: flexor/extensor/abdominal strengthening ▓ Durable medical equipment/offloading (walker/cane) ▓ Modalities (heat, ice, iontophoresis) ▓ Acupuncture ▓ OMT/manual therapy ▓ Physical therapy, aquatherapy ▓ Oral analgesics (NSAIDS, acetaminophen) ▓ Opioid analgesics ▓ Intra-articular steroid hip injection

Treatment Considerations for Common Pain Presentations (*Continued*)

Presentation	Treatment Considerations
Shoulder	▪ Activity modification ▪ Home exercise program—Codman's, scapular stabilization, wall walking, cuff strengthening, theraband exercises ▪ Modalities (heat, ice, iontophoresis, ultrasound) ▪ Acupuncture ▪ OMT/manual therapy (adhesive capsulitis) ▪ Physical therapy, aquatherapy ▪ Oral analgesics (NSAIDs, acetaminophen) ▪ Topical analgesics ▪ Opioid analgesics ▪ Steroid injection (glenohumeral, acromioclavicular, subacromial) ▪ RF/pulsed RF of intra-articular surfaces ▪ Nerve block—suprascapular
Bursitis	▪ Activity modification (offloading, avoid aggravation activities) ▪ Anti-inflammatories/consider topicals ▪ Steroid injection ▪ Physical therapy (eg, stretch ITB for GTB, stretch hip extensors for ischial bursitis) ▪ Modalities (ice) ▪ Opiates
Abdomen—Stomach/ upper	▪ Diet modification ▪ Antidepressants ▪ Anticholinergics ▪ Antispasmodics/baclofen ▪ Opiates with caution ▪ Acupuncture ▪ TENS ▪ Celiac plexus block

Treatment Considerations for Common Pain Presentations (Continued)

Presentation	Treatment Considerations
Abdomen–Pancreas	▪ Diet modification ▪ Cholecystokinin receptor antagonists ▪ Opiates ▪ Anti-inflammatory drugs ▪ Endoscopy ▪ Celiac plexus block
Abdomen: Lower	▪ Diet modification ▪ Anti-inflammatory drugs ▪ Opiates ▪ Antispasmodics ▪ Acupuncture ▪ TENS ▪ Superior hypogastric nerve block ▪ Iliohypogastric, ilioinguinal nerve block
Pelvic pain	▪ Opioid analgesics ▪ Neuropathic analgesics ▪ Sympathetic meds (clonidine, tizanidine) ▪ Antispasmodics ▪ Anticonvulsants ▪ Vaginal or rectal suppositories (baclofen, gabapentin) ▪ Hormonal therapy ▪ Physical therapy/pelvic floor therapy ± botulinum toxin therapy ▪ Massage therapy ▪ Intravaginal trigger injections ▪ Acupuncture ▪ OMT/manual therapy ▪ Caudal ESI ▪ Ganglion impar block ▪ Pudendal nerve block ▪ Spinal cord stimulation

Treatment Considerations for Common Pain Presentations (Continued)

Presentation	Treatment Considerations
CRPS	▪ Steroids ▪ Calcium-regulating drugs (calcitonin) ▪ Anticonvulsants ▪ Baclofen ▪ Clonidine ▪ Spinal cord stimulation ▪ Physical therapy (desensitization) ▪ Cognitive behavior therapy ▪ NSAIDs ▪ Sodium channel blockers ▪ Calcium channel blockers ▪ Opiates ▪ Antidepressants ▪ NMDA receptor blockers ▪ Stellate ganglion block vs LSB ▪ Bier block ▪ TENS ▪ Intrathecal pump (baclofen)
Compression fracture pain	▪ Calcitonin nasal spray ▪ Bisphosphonates ▪ Anti-inflammatories ▪ Opiates ▪ Extension-based exercise program ▪ Neuropathic pain meds ▪ Custom TLSO ▪ Epidural injection ▪ Vertebroplasty/kyphoplasty

Treatment Considerations for Common Pain Presentations (Continued)

Presentation	Treatment Considerations
Prostate	▪ Alpha blockers ▪ Anti-inflammatory drugs ▪ Muscle relaxants ▪ Antidepressants (TCA, SNRI) ▪ Anticonvulsants ▪ Anticholinergics ▪ Antibiotics ▪ Opiates ▪ 5-alpha reductase inhibitors ▪ Biofeedback ▪ Superior hypogastric nerve block
Peripheral neuropathy	▪ NMDA antagonist ▪ Alpha 2 blockers ▪ Antidepressants (TCA, SNRI) ▪ Anticonvulsants ▪ Calcium channel blockers ▪ Sodium channel blockers ▪ Opiates ▪ Interlaminar or caudal epidurals ▪ Sympathetic blocks (lumbar versus stellate) ▪ Topicals (nitroglycerin spray, capsaisin, voltarin) ▪ Lidocaine patch ▪ TENS ▪ Spinal cord stimulation

Initial Consultation Template

Patient Name:
MR#:
Date of Service:
Referring Physician:

Dear Dr. **[Referring Physician]:**
Thank you for your kind referral for **[patient name]** who presents to our clinic as follows:

Chief Complaint: [in patient's own words].

History of the Present Illness: Mr/Mrs/Ms. **[patient name]** is a very pleasant XX old.**[male/female]** who presents with **[chief complaint]**. The pain is located **[location]** and radiates to **[radiation]**. The patient has been experiencing this pain for **[duration]**. The patient relates a history of **[inciting events, accidents]**. The pain onset was **[sudden/insidious]**.

The pain is **[constant/intermittent]** in nature and described as **[descriptors]**. The pain is rated **[X/10]** on a visual analog scale. Exacerbating factors include **[factors]**. Alleviating factors include **[factors]**. There is **[no/ positive]** exacerbation of pain with cough or sneeze. The patient relates that the pain has a % lower/upper extremity component and % low back/ neck component **[if applicable]**. There are **[no]** bowel or bladder changes. The patient **[denies/reports]** weakness, numbness, or other deficits.

Treatment History: Treatment history includes visits to professional caregivers such as **[physicians]**.

The patient has a history of **[radiological and laboratory tests]**. Medication history includes **[medications and outcomes]**. Interventional history includes **[interventions and outcomes]**.

Past Medical History:

Past Surgical History:

Allergies:

Current Medications:

Social History: The patient denies any history of tobacco, alcohol, or recreational drugs or any exposures to toxins or poisonous substances.

Initial Consultation Template (*Continued*)

Family History: Noncontributory. She/he denies any history of childhood emotional trauma or physical or sexual abuse.

Review of Systems: Constitutional: **[no problems]**. Eyes: **[no problems]**. ENT: **[no problems]**. Cardiovascular: **[no problems]**. Respiratory: **[no problems]**. GI: **[no problems]**. GU: **[no problems]**. Musculoskeletal: **[see HPI]**. Skin/breast: **[no problems]**. Neurological: **[no problems]**. Psychiatric: **[no problems]**. Hematological/lymphatic: **[no problems]**. Allergic/immunologic: **[no problems]**. Endocrine: **[no problems]**. Constipation: **[none]**. Sedation: **[none]**. Pruritus: **[none]**. Sexual dysfunction: **[none]**.

PHYSICAL EXAMINATION:
Vital Signs:
General Appearance:
Cardiovascular: No pedal edema or varicosities are noted. Arterial strength is 2+ at the bilateral radial, brachial, popliteal, and dorsalis pedis arteries. Carotid amplitude and duration are normal without bruits. Lymphatic: There are no palpable nodes in the neck, axilla, or groin.

MUSCULOSKELETAL EXAMINATION:

Head and Neck:
Inspection of the neck reveals a **[supple, non-tender]** cervical spine **[with/without]** pain on palpation of the cervical facets **[at the XX level]**.

There is no frontal or maxillary sinus tenderness. There is no significant nasal congestion. There is no temporomandibular joint (TMJ) clicking or subluxation; there is no TMJ pain.

There is no pain on palpation of the bilateral greater occipital tuberosities and lesser occipital grooves.

Range of motion of the cervical spine reveals **[intact]** cervical flexion, extension, lateral rotation, and bending. There are **[no]** palpable tender or trigger points in the bilateral trapezii, paraspinal or parascapular musculature. Head and neck strength are within normal limits.
[For chief complaint of HA, please include cranial nerve exam.]

Lumbar Spine:
Station evaluation reveals: _____.

Inspection of the lumbar spine, ribs, and pelvis reveals **[no]** scoliosis and **[no]** pectus.

Palpation of the thoracic and lumbar facets and lumbar intervertebral spaces reveals **[no]** pain **[at the XX levels]**.

Initial Consultation Template (Continued)

There are **[no]** step-offs noted.

Range of motion of the lumbar spine reveals **[intact]** lumbar flexion, extension, and lateral bending. Lumbar extension and rotation (Kemp's Test) does **[not]** reproduce the patient's typical pain.

There are **[no]** palpable tender or trigger points in any of the muscles of the low back. Strength and tone of the lumbar musculature is **[normal]**. Palpation of the bilateral sacroiliac joints at the level of the posterior superior iliac spine (PSIS) reveals **[no]** pain. Patrick/FABER's test is **[negative/positive]** bilaterally. Internal rotation of the hips is intact and FAIR test is **[negative]** bilaterally. There does **[not]** appear to be any leg length discrepancy.

Shoulders: Inspection of the shoulders reveals **[no]** atrophy and **[no]** scapular dyskinesis. Palpation of the shoulders reveals **[no]** tenderness at the sternal notch, sternoclavicular joint, clavicle, acromioclavicular joint, and the biceps tendon. Range of motion of the shoulder reveals **[intact]** abduction, flexion, extension, and internal and external rotation. **[Negative/positive]** Neer, Hawkins, Empty Can, Speed's, Scarf test bilaterally. There is **[no]** evidence of dislocation on apprehension test bilaterally.

Knee: Inspection of the knees reveals **[normal]** varus and valgus alignment of the knee and **[normal]** assignment of the patella. There is **[no]** visible joint effusion. Palpation of the knees reveals no tenderness at the quadriceps tendon, patellar tendon, iliotibial band, pes anserinus bursa, or the medial and lateral joint lines. Range of motion of the knee reveals **[intact]** flexion and extension with **[no]** crepitus. **[Negative/positive]** patellar grind, Lachman's, anterior/posterior drawer, and McMurray tests. There is no laxity with varus or valgus stress.

Abdomen: Bowel sounds are **[normal/hypoactive]**. There is **[no]** tenderness to light/deep palpation. There is **[no]** organomegaly.

Pelvis: Inspection of the genitalia reveals **[no]** erythema or lesions. A bimanual examination reveals **[no]** pain on moving cervix. There is **[no]** adnexal tenderness. Sensation is **[intact/diminished]** to the iliohypogastric, ilioinguinal, genitofemoral, and lateral femoral cutaneous nerve distribution.

Initial Consultation Template (Continued)

Extremities: Examination of the bilateral lower extremities reveals **[no]** edema. Distal pulses are **[intact]**. Capillary refill is **[less than/greater than]** 5 seconds.

Skin: Inspection of the head, neck, trunk, and extremities is **[normal]**.

Neurologic: Coordination testing by finger-to-nose is **[within normal limits]**.

Deep tendon reflexes are **[0–4]** at the bilateral biceps, triceps, brachioradialis, patellar, and Achilles tendons. There are **[negative]** bilateral modified Hoffman responses and **[downgoing]** plantar reflexes. There is **[no]** clonus bilaterally.

Motor strength is:
[X/5] to the bilateral shoulder abductors
[X/5] to the bilateral elbow flexors
[X/5] to the bilateral elbow extensors
[X/5] to the bilateral wrist extensors
[X/5] to the bilateral wrist flexors
[X/5] to the bilateral hand grip
[X/5] to the bilateral abductor pollicis brevis (APB),
[X/5] to the bilateral finger interossei (abductors), **[X/5]** to the bilateral hip flexors, and
[X/5] to the bilateral knee extensors, **[X/5]** to the bilateral knee flexors,
[X/5] to the bilateral ankle dorsiflexors
[X/5] to the bilateral extensor hallicus longus
[X/5] to the bilateral toe flexors
[X/5] to the bilateral ankle plantar-flexors.

[Sensation is [intact/diminished] to pinprick in all dermatomes]: [from C5 to T2 bilaterally].
Sensation is **[intact/diminished]** to pinprick in all dermatomes: from L1 to S2 bilaterally.
Spurling test is **[negative/positive]** bilaterally.
Straight leg raising is **[negative/positive]** at **[X]** degrees bilaterally.
(Reverse straight leg raising is **[negative/positive]** bilaterally).
(Slump testing is **[negative/positive]** bilaterally).

Initial Consultation Template (*Continued*)

Gait evaluation reveals **[that the patient is able to heel, toe, and tandem walk appropriately without difficulties]. [The patient was also asked to do single leg stance lifts to better target any potential ankle plantar-flexor weakness. This was executed without difficulty bilaterally.]**

Diagnostic Data:

Impression:
1. **[diagnosis]**; 2. **[diagnosis]**; 3. **[diagnosis]**

Plan: Mr/Mrs/Ms. **[patient name]** is a **[XX]** old **[male/female]** who presents with **[chief complaint]**. Based on the patient's history, physical examination, and review of the available radiological imaging data...

Other diagnoses to be considered are...

To this effect, we recommend ... **[interventions/medications with exact dose/therapy/rehab/follow-up]**.

Please do not hesitate to contact us for any questions regarding the care of our mutual patient. And again, we thank you for this kind referral.
Rx Given: [medication/dose/sig/max per day/#dispensed]

Follow-Up Visit Template

Patient Name:
MR#:
Date of Service:
Referring Physician:

Chief Complaint: [in patient's own words].

History of the Present Illness: Mr/Mrs/Ms **[patient name]** is a very pleasant **[XX]** old **[male/female]** who presents with **[chief complaint]**. He/she was last seen on **[date]** at which time he/she had **[interventions, started on new medications, etc]**. He/she responded to this treatment with **[decrease in pain, no change in pain]**.

Currently, the pain is located **[location]** and radiates to **[radiation]**. The pain is **[constant/intermittent]** in nature and described as **[descriptors]**. The pain is rated X/10 on a visual analog scale. Exacerbating factors include **[factors]**. Alleviating factors include **[factors]**. There is **[no/positive]** exacerbation of pain with cough or sneeze. The patient relates that the pain has a % lower/upper extremity component and % low back/neck component **[if applicable]**. There are **[no]** bowel or bladder changes.

Current Medications: [including how taken; PRN use per day]

Review of Systems: The patient reports **[no]** nausea/vomiting/diarrhea/constipation/difficulty breathing/difficulty staying awake/or pruritus.

Medical History and Social History Update:
[These were reviewed with the patient: there is no new history to report]

PHYSICAL EXAMINATION:
Vital Signs:
General Appearance: [well groomed/disheveled/etc.]

Musculoskeletal Examination [only execute applicable regional PE]:

Head and Neck: Inspection of the neck reveals a **[supple, non-tender]** cervical spine **[with/without]** pain on palpation of the cervical facets **[at the XX level]**.

There is no frontal or maxillary sinus tenderness. There is no significant nasal congestion. There is no temporomandibular joint (TMJ) clicking or subluxation; there is no TMJ pain.

There is no pain on palpation of the bilateral greater occipital tuberosities and lesser occipital grooves.

Follow-Up Visit Template (Continued)

Range of motion of the cervical spine reveals **[intact]** cervical flexion, extension, lateral rotation and bending. There are **[no]** palpable tender or trigger points in the bilateral trapezii, paraspinal, or parascapular musculature. **[For chief complaint of HA, please include CN exam: Cranial Nerves II–XII are intact.]**

Lumbar Spine:
Station evaluation reveals: _____.

Inspection of the lumbar spine, ribs, and pelvis reveals **[no]** scoliosis and **[no]** pectus.

Palpation of the thoracic and lumbar facets and lumbar intervertebral spaces reveals **[no]** pain.

There are **[no]** step-offs noted.

Range of motion of the lumbar spine reveals **[intact]** lumbar flexion, extension, and lateral bending. Lumbar extension and rotation (Kemp's Test) does **[not]** reproduce the patient's typical pain.

There are **[no]** palpable tender or trigger points in any of the muscles of the low back. Strength and tone of the lumbar musculature is **[normal]**.

Palpation of the bilateral sacroiliac joints reveals **[no]** pain. Patrick/ FABER's test is **[negative/positive]** bilaterally. Internal rotation of the hips is **[intact]** and FAIR test is **[negative]** bilaterally. There does **[not]** appear to be any leg length discrepancy.

Shoulders: Inspection of the shoulders reveals **[no]** atrophy and **[no]** scapular dyskinesis. Palpation of the shoulders reveals **[no]** tenderness at the sternal notch, sternoclavicular joint, clavicle, acromioclavicular joint, and the biceps tendon. Range of motion of the shoulder reveals **[intact]** abduction, flexion, extension, and internal and external rotation. **[Negative/positive]** Neer, Hawkins, Empty Can, Speed's, and Scarf test bilaterally. There is **[no]** evidence of dislocation on apprehension test bilaterally.

Knee: Inspection of the knees reveals **[normal]** varus and valgus alignment of the knee and **[normal]** assignment of the patella. There is **[no]** visible joint effusion. Palpation of the knees reveals no tenderness at the quadriceps tendon, patellar tendon, iliotibial band, pes anserinus bursa, or the medial and lateral joint lines. Range of motion of the knee reveals **[intact]** flexion and extension with **[no]** crepitus. **[Negative/positive]** patellar grind, Lachman's, anterior/posterior drawer, and McMurray tests. There is no laxity with varus or valgus stress.

Follow-Up Visit Template *(Continued)*

Abdomen: Bowel sounds are **[normal/hypoactive]**. There is **[no]** tenderness to light/deep palpation. There is **[no]** organomegaly.

Pelvic: Inspection of the genitalia reveals **[no]** erythema or lesions. A bimanual examination reveals **[no]** pain on moving cervix. There is **[no]** adnexal tenderness. Sensation is **[intact/diminished]** to the iliohypogastric, ilioinguinal, genitofemoral, and lateral femoral cutaneous nerve distribution.

Extremities: Examination of the bilateral lower extremities reveals **[no]** edema. Distal pulses are **[intact]**. Capillary refill is **[less than/greater than]** 5 seconds.

Neurolgic: Coordination testing by finger-to-nose is **[within normal limits]**. Deep tendon reflexes are **[0–4]** at the bilateral biceps, triceps, brachioradialis, patellar, and Achilles tendons. There are **[negative]** bilateral modified Hoffman responses and **[downgoing]** plantar reflexes. There is **[no]** clonus bilaterally.

Motor strength is:
[X/5] to the bilateral shoulder abductors
[X/5] to the bilateral elbow flexors
[X/5] to the bilateral elbow extensors
[X/5] to the bilateral wrist extensors
[X/5] to the bilateral wrist flexors
[X/5] to the bilateral hand grip
[X/5] to the bilateral abductor pollicis brevis (APB)
[X/5] to the bilateral finger interossei (abductors)

[X/5] to the bilateral hip flexors
[X/5] to the bilateral knee extensors
[X/5] to the bilateral knee flexors
[X/5] to the bilateral ankle dorsiflexors
[X/5] to the bilateral extensor hallicus longus
[X/5] to the bilateral toe flexors
[X/5] to the bilateral ankle plantar-flexors

Follow-Up Visit Template (Continued)

Sensation is **[intact/diminished]** to pinprick in all dermatomes: from C5 to T2 bilaterally.

Sensation is **[intact/diminished]** to pinprick in all dermatomes: from L1 to S2 bilaterally.

Spurling test is **[negative/positive]** bilaterally.

Straight leg raising is **[negative/positive]** at **[X]** degrees bilaterally. (Reverse straight leg raising is **[negative/positive]** bilaterally.) (Slump testing is **[negative/positive]** bilaterally.)

Gait evaluation reveals **[that the patient is able to heel, toe, and tandem walk appropriately without difficulties].**

Signs of aberrant behavior are **[absent]**.

Impression:
1. **[diagnosis]**
2. **[diagnosis]**

Plan:

Mr/Mrs/Ms. **[patient name]** is a XX old **[male/female]** who is followed in our clinic for **[chief complaint]** ...
To this effect, we currently recommend... **[interventions/medications with exact dose/therapy/rehab/follow-up]**

Rx Given: [medication/dose/sig/max per day/#dispensed]

Interventional Procedure Templates

Trigger Point Injection

Patient Name:

MR#:

Date of Procedure:

Preoperative Diagnosis: Myalgia/Myositis 729.1

Postoperative Diagnosis: Myalgia/Myositis

Operation Title:

1) Trigger Point Injection

Attending Physician:

Assistant Physician:

Anesthesia: Local

Indications: The patient is a **[age]** old **[male/female]** with a diagnosis of myalgia/myositis. This is the **[x]** injection of **[#]**. **[The patient had [X]% relief from the previous injection.]** The patient's history and physical exam have been reviewed. The risks, benefits, and alternatives to the procedure have been discussed, and all questions have been answered to the patient's satisfaction. The patient agreed to proceed and a written informed consent was obtained.

Procedure in Detail: The patient was placed in a **[sitting/standing/ prone/ supine]** position. The area(s) of myofascial tightness was/were marked with the patient's assistance to localize the trigger points. The trigger points(s) was/were noted to be in the **[medial/lateral/superior/ inferior] [muscle: trapezius, gluteus maximus, L5 paraspinal, etc.]** These areas were then cleansed with alcohol × 3. A 1.25 inch 27-gauge needle attached to a 5 mL syringe filled with 5 mL 1% lidocaine was then inserted into the first marked trigger point area as the skin and subcutaneous tissues were lifted away from the body. Extensive dry needling was performed; each time a catch was felt with the needle, aspiration was performed and noted to be negative, and approximately 1 mL of 1% lidocaine was injected. The needle was then removed. The patient's **[back/neck/shoulder/etc.]** was then cleansed and a bandage was placed over the site of needle insertion. Deep tissue massage was then performed. The same procedure was repeated at the other marked trigger point locations.

The total volume of local anesthetic used was **[X mL]**.

Disposition: The patient tolerated the procedure well, and there were no apparent complications. **[Postoperative Plan Is ...]**

Greater Occipital Block

Patient Name: MR#:
Date of Procedure:
Preoperative Diagnosis: Occipital Neuralgia 723.8
Postoperative Diagnosis: Occipital Neuralgia
Operation Title:

1) **[Right/Left]** Greater Occipital Nerve Block
2) **[Right/Left]** Lesser Occipital Nerve Block

Attending Physician:
Assistant Physician:
Anesthesia: Local

Indications: The patient is a **[age]** old **[male/female]** with a diagnosis of Occipital Neuralgia. This is the **[x]** injection of **[#]**. **[The patient had [X]% relief from the previous injection.]** The patient's history and physical exam have been reviewed. The risks, benefits, and alternatives to the procedure have been discussed, and all questions have been answered to the patient's satisfaction. The patient agreed to proceed and written informed consent was obtained.

Procedure in Detail: The patient was placed in a sitting position with the neck in forward flexion. The occipital artery was palpated and the point of maximal tenderness, medial to the artery, was marked. This area was cleansed with alcohol times three. A 1.25 inch 27-gauge needle attached to a 5 mL syringe was then inserted into the scalp. After the occiput is encountered, the needle is withdrawn slightly, negative aspiration is elicited, and a subcutaneous depot of **[1 mL]** of a solution containing **[40 mg triamcinolone and 3 mL 1% lidocaine]** is injected. The needle was then removed.

[The point of maximal tenderness in the vicinity of the lesser occipital nerve, approximately 3 cm lateral to the occipital protuberance, is marked. This area is cleansed with alcohol times three. A 1.25 inch 27-gauge needle attached to a 5 mL syringe was then inserted into the scalp. After the occiput is encountered, the needle is withdrawn slightly, negative aspiration is elicited, and a depot of **[1 mL]** of a solution containing **[40 mg triamcinolone and 3 mL 1% lidocaine]** was injected in a fanning technique. The needle was then removed.]

The patient's head was cleansed and a bandage was placed over the site(s) of needle insertion.

[The same procedure was repeated on the opposite side.]

Disposition: The patient tolerated the procedure well, and there were no apparent complications. **[POSTOPERATIVE PLAN IS ...]**

.

Occipital Anatomy

Identify the occipital protuberance medially and the mastoid process laterally. The greater occipital nerve should lie on the medial third between these two areas, along the superior nuchal line and medial to the occipital artery. The lesser occipital nerve lies at the junction of the middle and outer third of a line between the occipital protuberance as the mastoid process. Inject into the subcutaneous tissue over the occipital bone. Inject diffusely, trying to distribute the medication in as large an area as possible. If the needle contacts the nerve, the patient may feel paresthesias in the distribution of the nerve. Do not inject into the nerve; withdraw the needle slightly. Always aspirate before injecting to ensure that you are not in the posterior occipital artery because this runs adjacent to the nerve. Do not inject forcefully because it is a fixed space and nerve trauma may result. Inject slowly.

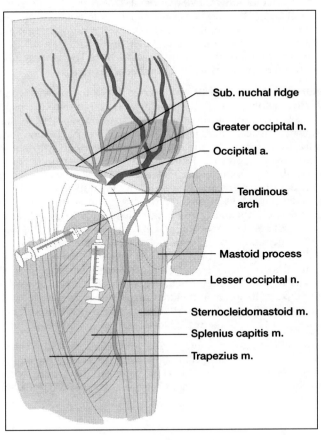

Lumbar Epidural Steroid Injection (ESI)

Patient Name: MR#: Date of Procedure:
Preoperative Diagnosis: **[Lumbar Radiculopathy/Spinal Stenosis]**
Postoperative Diagnosis: **[Lumbar Radiculopathy/Spinal Stenosis]**

Operation Title:
1) **[XX-XX]** Lumbar Epidural Steroid Injection (Interlaminar);
2) Intraoperative Fluoroscopy; 3) **[IV Conscious Sedation]**

Attending Physician:
Assistant Physician:
Anesthesia: Local **[and conscious sedation with Versed X mg and Fentanyl XX mcg]**

Indications: The patient is a **[age]** old **[male/female]** with a diagnosis of **[lumbar radiculopathy/spinal stenosis]**. This is the **[x]** injection of **[#]**. **[The patient had [X]% relief from the previous injection.]** The patient's history and physical exam have been reviewed. The risks, benefits, and alternatives to the procedure have been discussed, and all questions have been answered to the patient's satisfaction. The patient agreed to proceed and written informed consent was obtained.

Procedure in Detail: [An IV was started while the patient was in the preoperative holding area.] The patient was brought into the procedure room and placed in the prone position on the fluoroscopy table. Standard monitors were placed, and vital signs were observed throughout the procedure. The area of the lumbar spine was prepped with chloroprep times three and draped in a sterile manner. The **[XX–XX]** interspace was identified and marked under AP fluoroscopy. The skin and subcutaneous tissues in the area were anesthetized with 1% lidocaine. A **[XX]**-gauge Tuohy epidural needle was directed toward the interspace under fluoroscopic guidance until the ligamentum flavum was engaged. From this point, a loss of resistance technique with a glass syringe and **[saline/air]** was used to identify entrance of the needle into the epidural space. Once a good loss of resistance was obtained, negative aspiration was confirmed and 1 mL of contrast solution was injected. An appropriate epidurogram was noted. Then, after negative aspiration, a solution consisting of **[20 mg dexamethasone]** and **[4 mL]** preservative-free saline was easily injected. The needle was removed with a saline flush. The patient's back was cleaned and a bandage was placed over the site of needle insertion.

Disposition: The patient tolerated the procedure well, and there were no apparent complications. Vital signs remained stable throughout the procedure. The patient was taken to the recovery area where written discharge instructions for the procedure were given. **[POSTOP PLAN IS ...]**

Caudal ESI

Patient Name: MR#: Date of Procedure:
Preoperative Diagnosis: **[Lumbosacral Radiculopathy/Spinal Stenosis]**
Postoperative Diagnosis: **[Lumbosacral Radiculopathy/ Spinal Stenosis]**

Operation Title:
1) Caudal Epidural Steroid Injection; 2) Intraoperative Fluoroscopy;
3) **[IV Conscious Sedation]**

Attending Physician:
Assistant Physician:
Anesthesia: Local **[and conscious sedation with Versed X mg and Fentanyl XX mcg]**

Indications: The patient is a **[age]** old **[male/female]** with a diagnosis of **[Lumbosacral radiculopathy/spinal stenosis]**. This is the **[x]** injection of **[#]**. **[The patient had [X]% relief from the previous injection.]** The patient's history and physical exam have been reviewed. The risks, benefits, and alternatives to the procedure have been discussed, and all questions have been answered to the patient's satisfaction. The patient agreed to proceed and a written informed consent was obtained.

Procedure in Detail: [An IV was started while the patient was in the preoperative holding area.] The patient was brought into the procedure room and placed in the prone position on the fluoroscopy table. Standard monitors were placed, and vital signs were observed throughout the procedure. The area of the sacrum was prepped with chloroprep times three and draped in a sterile manner. The sacral hiatus was identified and marked under lateral fluoroscopy. The skin and subcutaneous tissues in the area were anesthetized with 1% lidocaine. A **[18-gauge Tuohy epidural]** needle was directed under fluoroscopic guidance until the epidural space was entered. **[An epidural catheter was then threaded superiorly until the tip of the catheter was noted to be at the XX vertebral level.]** Negative aspiration was confirmed and 1 mL of contrast solution was injected. An appropriate epidurogram was noted. Then, after negative aspiration, a solution consisting of **[20 mg dexamethasone]** and **[4 mL]** preservative-free saline was easily injected. The needle was removed with a saline flush. The patient's back was cleaned and a bandage was placed over the site of needle insertion.

Disposition: The patient tolerated the procedure well, and there were no apparent complications. Vital signs remained stable throughout the procedure. The patient was taken to the recovery area where written discharge instructions for the procedure were given. **[POSTOP PLAN IS ....]**

LumbarTransforaminal ESI: AP Approach
Patient Name: MR#: Date of Procedure:
Preoperative Diagnosis: **[Lumbar Radiculopathy]**
Postoperative Diagnosis: **[Lumbar Radiculopathy]**

Operation Title:
1) **XX** Transforaminal Epidural Steroid Injection; 2) Intraoperative
Fluoroscopy; 3) **[IV Conscious Sedation]**

Attending Physician:
Assistant Physician:
Anesthesia: Local **[and conscious sedation with Versed X mg and Fentanyl XX mcg]**

Indications: The patient is a **[age]** old **[male/female]** with a diagnosis of **[lumbar radiculopathy]**. This is the **[x]** injection of **[#]**. **[The patient had [X]% relief from the previous injection.]** The patient's history and physical exam have been reviewed. The risks, benefits, and alternatives to the procedure have been discussed, and all questions have been answered to the patient's satisfaction. The patient agreed to proceed and a written informed consent was obtained.

Procedure in Detail: [An IV was started while the patient was in the preoperative holding area.] The patient was brought into the procedure room and placed in the prone position on the fluoroscopy table. Standard monitors were placed, and vital signs were observed throughout the procedure. The area of the lumbar spine was prepped with chloroprep times three and draped in a sterile manner. The **[XX]** vertebral body was identified and marked under AP fluoroscopy. The skin and subcutaneous tissues in the area were anesthetized with 1% lidocaine. A 25-gauge 3.5 inch needle was directed toward the neuroforamen at the juncture of the transverse process and lateral border of the inferior laminae. The latter part of needle placement was guided by fluoroscopy in the lateral view until the needle tip was seen to enter the posterior epidural space. Negative aspiration was confirmed and 1 mL of contrast solution was injected. An appropriate epidurogram was noted. Then, after negative aspiration, a solution consisting of **[10 mg dexamethasone]** and **[1 mL]** preservative-free saline was easily injected. The needle was removed with a saline flush. The patient's back was cleaned and a bandage was placed over the site of needle insertion.

LumbarTransforaminal ESI: AP Approach (*Continued*)

[The right/left S1 foramen was identified and the 2 o'clock/10 o'clock position was marked. The skin and subcutaneous tissues in the area were anesthetized with 1% lidocaine. A 25-gauge 3.5 inch needle was then directed toward the target point under fluoroscopy until bone was contacted. The needle was then walked off inferiorly until the neuroforamen was entered. A lateral fluoroscopic view was then used to place the needle tip in the middle of the foramen.]

Negative aspiration was confirmed and 1 mL of contrast was injected at each level. Appropriate neurograms were observed under AP fluoroscopy. Then, again after negative fluoroscopy, a solution containing **[10 mg dexamethasone]** and **[1 mL]** preservative-free saline was easily injected. The needle was removed with a saline flush. The patient's back was cleaned and a bandage was placed over the site(s) of needle insertion.

Disposition: The patient tolerated the procedure well, and there were no apparent complications. Vital signs remained stable throughout the procedure. The patient was taken to the recovery area where written discharge instructions for the procedure were given. **[POSTOP PLAN IS ...]**

Lumbar Transforaminal ESI: Oblique Approach

Patient Name: MR#:
Date of Procedure:
Preoperative Diagnosis: **[Lumbar Radiculopathy]**
Postoperative Diagnosis: **[Lumbar Radiculopathy]**

Operation Title:
1) **[XX]** Transforaminal Epidural Steroid Injection; 2) Intraoperative
Fluoroscopy; 3) **[IV Conscious Sedation]**

Attending Physician:
Assistant Physician:
Anesthesia: Local **[and conscious sedation with Versed X mg and Fentanyl XX mcg]**

Indications: The patient is a **[age]** old **[male/female]** with a diagnosis of **[lumbar radiculopathy]**. This is the **[x]** injection of **[#]**. **[The patient had [X]% relief from the previous injection.]** The patient's history and physical exam have been reviewed. The risks, benefits, and alternatives to the procedure have been discussed, and all questions have been answered to the patient's satisfaction. The patient agreed to proceed and written informed consent was obtained.

Procedure in Detail: [An IV was started while the patient was in the preoperative holding area.] The patient was brought into the procedure room and placed in the prone position on the fluoroscopy table. Standard monitors were placed, and vital signs were observed throughout the procedure. The area of the lumbar spine was prepped with chloroprep times three and draped in a sterile manner. The **[XX]** vertebral body was identified and marked under AP fluoroscopy. An oblique view to the **[right/left]** was obtained to better visualize the inferior junction of the pedicle and transverse process. The 6 o'clock position below the pedicle was marked.

The skin and subcutaneous tissues in the area were anesthetized with saline flush. A 25-gauge 3.5 inch needle was directed toward the targeted point under fluoroscopy until the bone was contacted. The needle was then walked off inferiorly until the neuroforamen was entered. A lateral fluoroscopic view was then used to place the needle tip at the 10 o'clock position of the foramen.

Lumbar Transforaminal ESI: Oblique Approach (*Continued*)

[The right/left S1 foramen was identified and the 2 o'clock/10 o'clock position was marked. The skin and subcutaneous tissues in the area were anesthetized with 1% lidocaine. A 25-gauge 3.5 inch needle was then directed toward the target point under fluoroscopy until bone was contacted. The needle was then walked off inferiorly until the neuroforamen was entered. A lateral fluoroscopic view was then used to place the needle tip in the middle of the foramen.]

Negative aspiration was confirmed and 1 mL of contrast was injected at each level. Appropriate neurograms were observed under AP fluoroscopy. Then, again after negative aspiration, a solution containing **[10 mg dexamethasone]** and **[1 mL]** preservative-free saline was easily injected. The needle was removed with a saline flush. The patient's back was cleaned and a bandage was placed over the site(s) of needle insertion.

Disposition: The patient tolerated the procedure well, and there were no apparent complications. Vital signs remained stable throughout the procedure. The patient was taken to the recovery area where written discharge instructions for the procedure were given. **[POSTOP PLAN IS ...]**

Cervical Selective Nerve Root

Patient Name: MR#: Date of Procedure:
Preoperative Diagnosis: **[Cervical Radiculopathy]**
Postoperative Diagnosis: **[Cervical Radiculopathy]**

Operation Title:
1) **[XX-XX [Right/Left]]** Cervical Selective Nerve Root Block; 2) Intraoperative Fluoroscopy; 3) **[IV Conscious Sedation]**

Attending Physician:
Assistant Physician:
Anesthesia: Local **[and conscious sedation with ...]**

Indications: The patient is a **[age]** old **[male/female]** with a diagnosis of **[cervical radiculopathy]**. The patient's history and physical exam have been reviewed. The risks, benefits, and alternatives to the procedure have been discussed, and all questions have been answered to the patient's satisfaction. The patient agreed to proceed and written informed consent was obtained.

Procedure in Detail: [An IV was started while the patient was in the preoperative holding area.] The patient was brought into the procedure room and placed in the supine position on the fluoroscopy table. Standard monitors were placed, and vital signs were observed throughout the procedure. The area of the cervical spine was prepped with chloroprep times three and draped in a sterile manner. The **[XX-XX]** interspace was identified and marked under AP fluoroscopy. A far oblique view to the **[right/left]** was obtained to better visualize the neuroforamen. A position was marked at the superoposterior edge of the neuroformen. Palpation confirmed a lack of proximity to any vascular structures. The skin and subcutaneous tissues in the area were anesthetized with 1% lidocaine. A 22-gauge 3.5 inch needle was directed toward the targeted point under fluoroscopy until bone was contacted. The needle was then retracted 1 mm. After negative aspiration was confirmed, 1 mL of contrast solution was injected. An appropriate neurogram was noted.

Then, after negative aspiration, a solution consisting of **[1 mL]** 0.25% bupivacaine was easily injected. The patient's back was cleaned and a bandage was placed over the site of needle insertion.

Disposition: The patient tolerated the procedure well, and there were no apparent complications. Vital signs remained stable throughout the procedure. The patient was taken to the recovery area where written discharge instructions for the procedure were given. **[POSTOP PLAN IS ...]**

Cervical ESI

Patient Name: MR#: Date of Procedure:
Preoperative Diagnosis: **[Cervical Radiculopathy/Spinal Stenosis]**
Postoperative Diagnosis: **[Cervical Radiculopathy/Spinal Stenosis]**

Operation Title:
1) **[XX-XX]** Cervical Epidural Steroid Injection; 2) Intraoperative
Fluoroscopy; 3) **[IV Conscious Sedation]**

Attending Physician:
Assistant Physician:
Anesthesia: Local **[and conscious sedation with ...]**

Indications: The patient is a **[age]** old **[male/female]** with a diagnosis of
[cervical radiculopathy/spinal stenosis]. This is the **[x]** injection of **[#]**.
[The patient had [X]% relief from the previous injection.] The patient's
history and physical exam have been reviewed. The risks, benefits, and
alternatives to the procedure have been discussed, and all questions
have been answered to the patient's satisfaction. The patient agreed to
proceed and a written informed consent was obtained.

Procedure in Detail: **[An IV was started while the patient was in the
pre-operative holding area.]** The patient was brought into the procedure room and placed in the prone position on the fluoroscopy table.
Standard monitors were placed, and vital signs were observed throughout the procedure. The area of the cervical spine was prepped with
chloroprep times three and draped in a sterile manner. The **[XX-XX]**
interspace was identified and marked under AP fluoroscopy. The skin
and subcutaneous tissues in the area were anesthetized with 1% lidocaine. A 17-gauge Tuohy epidural needle was directed toward the interspace under fluoroscopic guidance until the superior border of the
inferior lamina was contacted. From this point, the needle was walked
off the lamina superiorly and a loss of resistance technique with a glass
syringe and saline was used to identify entrance of the needle into the
epidural space. Once a good loss of resistance was obtained, negative
aspiration was confirmed and 1 mL of contrast solution was injected. An
appropriate epidurogram was noted. Then, after negative aspiration, a
solution consisting of **[20 mg dexamethasone]** and **[4 mL]** preservative-
free saline was easily injected. The needle was removed with a saline
flush. The patient's back was cleaned and a bandage was placed over
the site of needle insertion.

Disposition: The patient tolerated the procedure well, and there were
no apparent complications. Vital signs remained stable throughout the
procedure. The patient was taken to the recovery area where written discharge instructions for the procedure were given. **[POSTOP PLAN IS ...]**

Thoracic ESI
Patient Name: MR#: Date of Procedure:
Preoperative Diagnosis: **[Thoracic Radiculopathy]**
Postoperative Diagnosis: **[Thoracic Radiculopathy]**

Operation Title:
1) **[XX-XX]** Thoracic Epidural Steroid Injection; 2) Intraoperative Fluoroscopy; 3) **[IV Conscious Sedation]**

Attending Physician:
Assistant Physician:
Anesthesia: Local **[and conscious sedation with ...]**

Indications: The patient is a **[age]** old **[male/female]** with a diagnosis of **[thoracic radiculopathy].** This is the **[x]** injection of **[#]**. **[The patient had [X]% relief from the previous injection.]** The patient's history and physical exam have been reviewed. The risks, benefits, and alternatives to the procedure have been discussed, and all questions have been answered to the patient's satisfaction. The patient agreed to proceed and written informed consent was obtained.

Procedure in Detail: [An IV was started while the patient was in the preoperative holding area.] The patient was brought into the procedure room and placed in the prone position on the fluoroscopy table. Standard monitors were placed, and vital signs were observed throughout the procedure. The area of the thoracic spine was prepped with chloroprep times three and draped in a sterile manner. The **[XX-XX]** interspace was identified and marked under AP fluoroscopy. The skin and subcutaneous tissues in the area were anesthetized with 1% lidocaine. A 17-gauge Tuohy epidural needle was directed toward the interspace under fluoroscopic guidance until the superior border of the inferior lamina was contacted. From this point, the needle was walked off the lamina superiorly and a loss of resistance technique with a glass syringe and saline was used to identify entrance of the needle into the epidural space. Once a good loss of resistance was obtained, negative aspiration was confirmed and 1 mL of contrast solution was injected. An appropriate epidurogram was noted. Then, after negative aspiration, a solution consisting of **[20 mg dexamethasone]** and **[4 mL]** preservative-free saline was easily injected. The needle was removed with a saline flush. The patient's back was cleaned and a bandage was placed over the site of needle insertion.

Disposition: The patient tolerated the procedure well, and there were no apparent complications. Vital signs remained stable throughout the procedure. The patient was taken to the recovery area where written discharge instructions for the procedure were given. **[POSTOP PLAN IS...]**

Lumbar Medial Branch Nerve Block (MBNB): AP Approach

Patient Name: MR#: Date of Procedure:
Preoperative Diagnosis: **[Lumbar Facet Arthropathy]**
Postoperative Diagnosis: **[Lumbar Facet Arthropathy]**

Operation Title:
1) **[XX]** Medial Branch Block; 2) Intraoperative Fluoroscopy; 3) **[IV Conscious Sedation]**

Attending Physician:
Assistant Physician:
Anesthesia: Local **[and conscious sedation with ...]**

Indications: The patient is a **[age]** old **[male/female]** with a diagnosis of **[lumbar facet arthropathy]**. This is the **[x]** injection of **[#]**. **[The patient had [X]% relief from the previous injection.]** The patient's history and physical exam have been reviewed. The risks, benefits, and alternatives to the procedure have been discussed, and all questions have been answered to the patient's satisfaction. The patient agreed to proceed and written informed consent was obtained.

Procedure in Detail: The patient was brought into the procedure room and placed in the prone position on the fluoroscopy table. Standard monitors were placed and vital signs were observed throughout the procedure. The area of the lumbar spine was prepped with chloroprep times three and draped in a sterile manner. AP fluoroscopy was used to identify and mark Barton's point at the **[XX-XX]** levels on the **[right/left]** side. **[The sacral ala and the 2 o'clock/10 o'clock position of the right/ left S1 foramen were identified and marked.]** The skin and subcutaneous tissues in these identified areas were anesthetized with 1% lidocaine. A 25-gauge 3.5 inch spinal needle was advanced toward each of these points under fluoroscopic guidance. Once bone was contacted, negative aspiration was confirmed and **[1 mL]** of **[0.5% bupivacaine]** was injected at each level.

[The same procedure was repeated on the opposite side.]

After the procedure was completed, the patient's back was cleaned and bandages were placed at the needle insertion sites.

Disposition: The patient tolerated the procedure well and there were no apparent complications. Vital signs remained stable throughout the procedure. The patient was taken to the recovery area where written discharge instructions for the procedure were given. **[POSTOP PLAN IS ...]**

Preop Exam: [XXXXX]
Postop Exam: [XXXX]. Postoperative pain relief **[was/was not]** significant.

Facet Innervation Anatomy

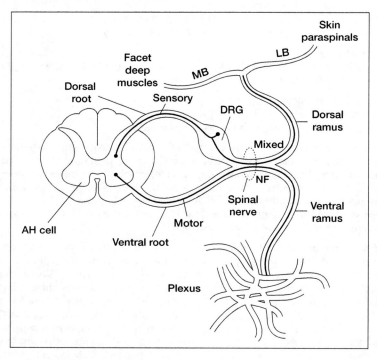

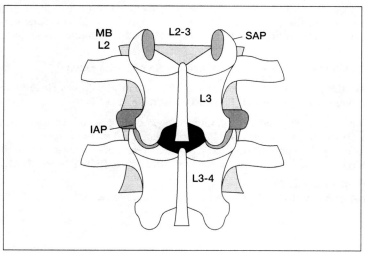

Lumbar MBNB: Oblique Approach

Patient Name: MR#: Date of Procedure:
Preoperative Diagnosis: [**Lumbar Facet Arthropathy**]
Postoperative Diagnosis: [**Lumbar Facet Arthropathy**]

Operation Title:
1) [**XX**] Medial Branch Block; 2) Intraoperative Fluoroscopy;
3) [**IV Conscious Sedation**]

Attending Physician:
Assistant Physician:
Anesthesia: Local [**and conscious sedation with ...**]

Indications: The patient is a [**age**] old [**male/female**] with a diagnosis of [**lumbar facet arthropathy**]. This is the [**x**] injection of [**#**]. [**The patient had [X]% relief from the previous injection.**] The patient's history and physical exam have been reviewed. The risks, benefits, and alternatives to the procedure have been discussed, and all questions have been answered to the patient's satisfaction. The patient agreed to proceed and a written informed consent was obtained.

Procedure in Detail: The patient was brought into the procedure room and placed in the prone position on the fluoroscopy table. Standard monitors were placed and vital signs were observed throughout the procedure. The area of the lumbar spine was prepped with chloroprep times three and draped in a sterile manner. AP and oblique fluoroscopy were used to identify and mark the junctions between the superior articular processes and transverse processes at the [**XX-XX**] levels on the [**right/left**] side. [**The sacral ala and the 2 o'clock/ 10 o'clock position of the right/left S1 foramen were identified and marked.**] The skin and subcutaneous tissues in these identified areas were anesthetized with 1% lidocaine. A 25-gauge 3.5 inch spinal needle was advanced toward each of these points under fluoroscopic guidance. Once bone was contacted, negative aspiration was confirmed and [**1 mL**] of [**0.5% bupivacaine**] was injected at each level. [**The same procedure was repeated on the opposite side.**] After the procedure was completed, the patient's back was cleaned and bandages were placed at the needle insertion sites.

Disposition: The patient tolerated the procedure well and there were no apparent complications. Vital signs remained stable throughout the procedure. The patient was taken to the recovery area where written discharge instructions for the procedure were given. [**POSTOP PLAN IS ...**]

Preop Exam: [XXXXX]
Postop Exam: [XXXX]. Postoperative pain relief [**was/was not**] significant.

Cervical MBNB: Lateral Approach

Patient Name: MR#: Date of Procedure:
Preoperative Diagnosis: **[Cervical Facet Arthropathy]**
Postoperative Diagnosis: **[Cervical Facet Arthropathy]**

Operation Title:
1) **[XX]** Medial Branch Block; 2) Intraoperative Fluoroscopy;
3) **[IV Conscious Sedation]**

Attending Physician:
Assistant Physician:
Anesthesia: Local **[and conscious sedation with ...]**

Indications: The patient is a **[age]** old **[male/female]** with a diagnosis of **[cervical facet arthropathy]**. This is the **[x]** injection of **[#]**. **[The patient had [X]% relief from the previous injection.]** The patient's history and physical exam have been reviewed. The risks, benefits, and alternatives to the procedure have been discussed, and all questions have been answered to the patient's satisfaction. The patient agreed to proceed and written informed consent was obtained.

Procedure in Detail: The patient was brought into the procedure room and placed in the **[supine]** position on the fluoroscopy table. Standard monitors were placed and vital signs were observed throughout the procedure. The area of the neck and cervical spine were prepped with chloroprep times three and draped in a sterile manner. Lateral fluoroscopy was used to identify the centroid positions of the mid-articular pillars of the **[XX-XX]** levels on the **[right/left]** side. The skin and subcutaneous tissues in these identified areas were anesthetized with 1% lidocaine. A 22-gauge. A 1.5 inch needle was advanced toward each of these points under fluoroscopic guidance. Once bone was contacted, negative aspiration was confirmed and **[0.5 mL]** of **[0.5% bupivacaine]** was injected at each level.

[The same procedure was repeated on the opposite side.]

After the procedure was completed, the patient's neck was cleaned and bandages were placed at the needle insertion sites.

Disposition: The patient tolerated the procedure well and there were no apparent complications. Vital signs remained stable throughout the procedure. The patient was taken to the recovery area where written discharge instructions for the procedure were given. **[POSTOP PLAN IS ...]**

Preop Exam: [XXXXX]
Postop Exam: [XXXX]. Postoperative pain relief **[was/was not]** significant.

Cervical MBNB: AP Approach

Patient Name: MR#: Date of Procedure:
Preoperative Diagnosis: **[Cervical Facet Arthropathy]**
Postoperative Diagnosis: **[Cervical Facet Arthropathy]**

Operation Title:
1) **[XX]** Medial Branch Block; 2) Intraoperative Fluoroscopy;
3) **[IV Conscious Sedation]**

Attending Physician:
Assistant Physician:
Anesthesia: Local **[and conscious sedation with ...]**

Indications: The patient is a **[age]** old **[male/female]** with a diagnosis of **[cervical facet arthropathy]**. This is the **[x]** injection of **[#]**. **[The patient had [X]% relief from the previous injection.]** The patient's history and physical exam have been reviewed. The risks, benefits, and alternatives to the procedure have been discussed, and all questions have been answered to the patient's satisfaction. The patient agreed to proceed and written informed consent was obtained.

Procedure in Detail: The patient was brought into the procedure room and placed in the supine position on the fluoroscopy table. Standard monitors were placed and vital signs were observed throughout the procedure. The area of the neck and cervical spine were prepped with chloroprep times three and draped in a sterile manner. AP fluoroscopy was used to identify the waists of the mid-articular pillars of the **[XX-XX]** levels on the **[right/left]** side. The skin and subcutaneous tissues in these identified areas were anesthetized with 1% lidocaine. A 22-gauge 1.5 inch needle was advanced toward each of these points under fluoroscopic guidance. Once bone was contacted, lateral fluoroscopic views were obtained and the needle was advanced to the centroid of the facets at each level. After negative aspiration was confirmed, **[0.5 mL]** of **[0.5% bupivacaine]** was injected at each level.

[The same procedure was repeated on the opposite side.]

After the procedure was completed, the patient's neck was cleaned and bandages were placed at the needle insertion sites.

Disposition: The patient tolerated the procedure well and there were no apparent complications. Vital signs remained stable throughout the procedure. The patient was taken to the recovery area where written discharge instructions for the procedure were given. **[POSTOP PLAN IS ...]**

Preop Exam: [XXXXX]
Postop Exam: [XXXX]. Postoperative pain relief **[was/was not]** significant.

Intercostal Nerve Block

Patient Name: MR#: Date of Procedure:
Preoperative Diagnosis: **[Intercostal Neuralgia]**
Postoperative Diagnosis: **[Intercostal Neuralgia]**

Operation Title:
1) **[XX, XX]** Intercostal Nerve Block(s);
2) Intraoperative Fluoroscopy; 3) **[IV Conscious Sedation]**

Attending Physician:
Assistant Physician:
Anesthesia: Local **[and conscious sedation with ...]**

Indications: The patient is a **[age]** old **[male/female]** with a diagnosis of **[intercostal neuralgia]**. This is the **[x]** injection of **[#]**. **[The patient had [X]% relief from the previous injection.]** The patient's history and physical exam have been reviewed. The risks, benefits, and alternatives to the procedure have been discussed, and all questions have been answered to the patient's satisfaction. The patient agreed to proceed and a written informed consent was obtained.

Procedure in Detail: [An IV was started while the patient was in the preoperative holding area.] The patient was brought into the procedure room and placed in the prone position on the fluoroscopy table. Standard monitors were placed, and vital signs were observed throughout the procedure. The area of the thoracic spine was prepped with chloroprep times three and draped in a sterile manner. The **[[right/left] T [X] - T [X]]** ribs were identified and the inferior margin at the angle of each rib was identified and marked under AP fluoroscopy. The skin and subcutaneous tissues in the area were anesthetized with 1% lidocaine. A **[22-gauge 1.5 inch]** needle was directed toward the inferior aspect of each rib under fluoroscopic guidance until the bone was engaged. From this point, the needle was walked off the rib inferiorly. Once negative aspiration was confirmed; 1 mL of contrast solution was injected. An appropriate spread of contrast was noted in the nerve sheath.

Then, after negative aspiration, **[1 mL]** of a solution containing **[3 mL 0.25% bupivacaine]** and **[40 mg triamcinolone]** was injected at each level (10 mg triamcinolone per level). The needle was removed with a saline flush. The patient's back was cleaned and bandages were placed over the sites of needle insertion.

Disposition: The patient tolerated the procedure well, and there were no apparent complications. Vital signs remained stable throughout the procedure. The patient was taken to the recovery area where written discharge instructions for the procedure were given. **[POSTOP PLAN IS ...]**

Intercostal Anatomy

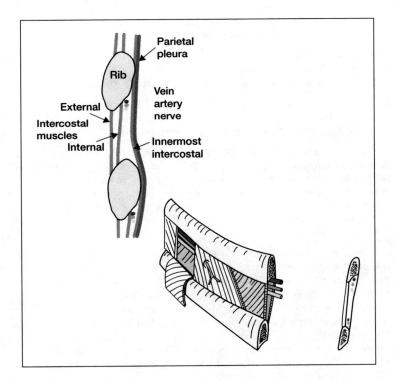

Sacroiliac Joint Injection
Patient Name: MR#: Date of Procedure:
Preoperative Diagnosis: **[Sacroiliac Dysfunction]**
Postoperative Diagnosis: **[Sacroiliac Dysfunction]**

Operation Title:
1) **[Right/Left]** Sacroiliac Joint Injection;
2) Intraoperative Fluoroscopy; 3) **[IV Conscious Sedation]**

Attending Physician:
Assistant Physician:
Anesthesia: Local **[and conscious sedation with ...]**

Indications: The patient is a **[age]** old **[male/female]** with a diagnosis of **[Sacroiliac dysfunction]**. This is the **[x]** injection of **[#]**. **[The patient had [X]% relief from the previous injection.]** The patient's history and physical exam have been reviewed. The risks, benefits, and alternatives to the procedure have been discussed, and all questions have been answered to the patient's satisfaction. The patient agreed to proceed and written informed consent was obtained.

Procedure in Detail: [An IV was started while the patient was in the pre-operative holding area.] The patient was brought into the procedure room and placed in the prone position on the fluoroscopy table. Standard monitors were placed, and vital signs were observed throughout the procedure. The area of the low back and upper buttock was prepped with chloroprep times three and draped in a sterile manner. The **[right/left]** sacroiliac joint was identified and marked under AP fluoroscopy. The fluoroscopic bean was then oblique until the anterior and posterior margins of the joint were aligned. The inferior margin of the joint was identified and marked. The skin and subcutaneous tissues in the area were anesthetized with 1% lidocaine. A 25-gauge 3.5 inch needle was directed toward the identified point under fluoroscopic guidance. Once the targeted point was reached and the joint space was entered, negative aspiration was confirmed and 1 mL of contrast solution was injected. An appropriate arthrogram was noted.

Then, after negative aspiration, a solution consisting of **[40 mg triamcinolone]** and **[1 mL]** preservative-free saline was easily injected. The needle was removed with a saline flush. The patient's back was cleaned and a bandage was placed over the site of needle insertion.

Disposition: The patient tolerated the procedure well, and there were no apparent complications. Vital signs remained stable throughout the procedure. The patient was taken to the recovery area where written discharge instructions for the procedure were given. **[POSTOP PLAN IS ...]**

Greater Trocanteric Bursa Injection

Patient Name: MR#: Date of Procedure:
Preoperative Diagnosis: **[Greater Trocanteric Bursitis]**
Postoperative Diagnosis: **[Greater Trocanteric Bursitis]**
Operation Title:

1) **[Right/Left]** Greater Trocanteric Bursa Injection;
2) Intraoperative Fluoroscopy; 3) **[IV Conscious Sedation]**

Attending Physician:
Assistant Physician:
Anesthesia: Local **[and conscious sedation with ...]**

Indications: The patient is a **[age]** old **[male/female]** with a diagnosis of **[Greater Trocanteric Bursitis]**. This is the **[x]** injection of **[#]**. **[The patient had [X]% relief from the previous injection.]** The patient's history and physical exam have been reviewed. The risks, benefits, and alternatives to the procedure have been discussed, and all questions have been answered to the patient's satisfaction. The patient agreed to proceed and written informed consent was obtained.

Procedure in Detail: The patient was brought into the procedure room and placed in the **[supine]** position on the fluoroscopy table. Standard monitors were placed, and vital signs were observed throughout the procedure. The area of the **[right/left]** greater trocanter was prepped with chloroprep times three and draped in a sterile manner. The **[right/left]** greater trocanter was identified under AP fluoroscopy and marked at a site just inferior to its greatest prominence. A lateral image was then obtained to check depth and the greater trocanter was again marked just inferior to its greatest prominence. A point of needle insertion was then chosen at the intersection of these two planes. The skin and subcutaneous tissues in this area were anesthetized with 1% lidocaine. A 25-gauge 3.5 inch needle was directed toward the identified point under fluoroscopic guidance. Once the bone was contacted, the needle was withdrawn slightly. After negative aspiration was confirmed and 1 mL of contrast solution was injected, an appropriate bursagram was noted.

Then, after negative aspiration, a solution consisting of **[40 mg triamcinolone]** and **[3 mL] [0.25% bupivacaine]** was easily injected. The needle was removed with a saline flush. The patient's leg was cleaned and a bandage was placed over the site of needle insertion.

Disposition: The patient tolerated the procedure well, and there were no apparent complications. Vital signs remained stable throughout the procedure. The patient was taken to the recovery area where written discharge instructions for the procedure were given. **[POSTOP PLAN IS ...]**

Piriformis Muscle Injection

Patient Name: MR#: Date of Procedure:
Preoperative Diagnosis: **[Piriformis Syndrome]**
Postoperative Diagnosis: **[Piriformis Syndrome]**

Operation Title:
1) **[Right/Left]** Piriformis Muscle Injection;
2) Intraoperative Fluoroscopy; 3) **[IV Conscious Sedation]**

Attending Physician:
Assistant Physician:
Anesthesia: Local **[and conscious sedation with ...]**

Indications: The patient is a **[age]** old **[male/female]** with a diagnosis of **[Right/Left]** **[Piriformis Syndrome]**. This is the **[x]** injection of **[#]**. **[The patient had [X]% relief from the previous injection.]** The patient's history and physical exam have been reviewed. The risks, benefits, and alternatives to the procedure have been discussed, and all questions have been answered to the patient's satisfaction. The patient agreed to proceed and written informed consent was obtained.

Procedure in Detail: The patient was brought into the procedure room and placed in the **[prone]** position on the fluoroscopy table. Standard monitors were placed, and vital signs were observed throughout the procedure. The area of the low back and buttock were prepped with chloroprep times three and draped in a sterile manner. The skin and subcutaneous tissues in this area were anesthetized with 1% lidocaine.

Under AP fluoroscopy, the **[11 o'clock/1 o'clock]** position on the **[right/left]** acetabular rim was identified and marked.

A 25-gauge 3.5 inch needle was directed toward the identified point under fluoroscopic guidance. Once the bone was contacted, the needle was withdrawn slightly. After negative aspiration was confirmed, 1 mL of contrast solution was injected and an appropriate outline of the piriformis muscle, in a vertical band, was observed without intravascular or epidural uptake.

Negative aspiration was again confirmed and **[40 mg depo-medrol]** with **[2 mL of 1% lidocaine and 1 mL of contrast]** was injected. The needle was removed with a saline flush. The patient's back was cleaned and a bandage was placed over the site of needle insertion.

Disposition: The patient tolerated the procedure well, and there were no apparent complications. Vital signs remained stable throughout the procedure. The patient was taken to the recovery area where written discharge instructions for the procedure were given. **[POSTOP PLAN IS ...]**

Intra-Articular Hip Injection

Patient Name: MR#: Date of Procedure:
Preoperative Diagnosis: **[Hip Osteoarthritis]**
Postoperative Diagnosis: **[Hip Osteoarthritis]**

Operation Title:
1) **[Right/Left]** Intra-Articular Hip Injection;
2) Intraoperative Fluoroscopy; 3) **[IV Conscious Sedation]**

Attending Physician:
Assistant Physician:
Anesthesia: Local **[and conscious sedation with ...]**

Indications: The patient is a **[age]** old **[male/female]** with a diagnosis of **[Right/Left]** **[Hip osteoarthritis and hip pain]**. This is the **[x]** injection of **[#]**. **[The patient had [X]% relief from the previous injection.]** The patient's history and physical exam have been reviewed. The risks, benefits, and alternatives to the procedure have been discussed, and all questions have been answered to the patient's satisfaction. The patient agreed to proceed and written informed consent was obtained.

Procedure in Detail: The patient was brought into the procedure room and placed in the **[lateral]** position on the fluoroscopy table. Standard monitors were placed, and vital signs were observed throughout the procedure. The areas of the bilateral femoral heads were aligned to overlap in the lateral view. The midpoint of the **[right/left]** femoral head was identified and marked. Under AP fluoroscopy, the femoral neck was then identified and marked. A point of needle insertion was then chosen at the intersection of these planes. This area was prepped with chloroprep times three and draped in a sterile manner. The skin and subcutaneous tissues in this area were anesthetized with 1% lidocaine. A 25-gauge 3.5 inch needle was directed toward the identified point under fluoroscopic guidance. Once the bone was contacted, the needle was withdrawn slightly. After negative aspiration was confirmed and 1 mL of contrast solution was injected. An appropriate arthrogram was noted.

Then, after negative aspiration, a solution consisting of **[40 mg triamcinolone]** and **[3 mL]** **[0.25% bupivacaine]** was easily injected. The needle was removed with a saline flush. The patient's leg was cleaned and a bandage was placed over the site of needle insertion.

Disposition: The patient tolerated the procedure well, and there were no apparent complications. Vital signs remained stable throughout the procedure. The patient was taken to the recovery area where written discharge instructions for the procedure were given. **[POSTOP PLAN IS ...]**

Intra-Articular Knee Injection

Patient Name: MR#: Date of Procedure:
Preoperative Diagnosis: **[Knee Osteoarthritis]**
Postoperative Diagnosis: **[Knee Osteoarthritis]**

Operation Title:
1) **[Right/Left]** Intra-Articular Knee Injection;
2) Intraoperative Fluoroscopy; 3) **[IV Conscious Sedation]**

Attending Physician:
Assistant Physician:

Indications: The patient is a **[age]** old **[male/female]** with a diagnosis of **[Right/Left]** **[knee osteoarthritis and knee pain]**. This is the **[x]** injection of **[#]**. **[The patient had [X]% relief from the previous injection.]** The patient's history and physical exam have been reviewed. The risks, benefits, and alternatives to the procedure have been discussed, and all questions have been answered to the patient's satisfaction. The patient agreed to proceed and written informed consent was obtained.

Procedure in Detail: The patient was brought into the procedure room and placed in the **[sitting]** position on the table. The **[right/left]** knee was placed in 90 degrees of flexion. The inferomedial border of the patella was palpated and marked for intra-articular access. The knee was prepped with chloroprep times three. The skin and subcutaneous tissues in this area were anesthetized with ethyl chloride spray. A 25-gauge 3.5 inch needle was directed toward the identified point in a superior trajectory until the femur was contacted in the posterior part of the joint space. Once the bone was contacted, the needle was withdrawn slightly. After negative aspiration was confirmed, a solution consisting of **[40 mg triamcinolone]** and **[3 mL]** **[0.25% bupivacaine]** was easily injected. The needle was removed with a saline flush. The patient's leg was cleaned and a bandage was placed over the site of needle insertion.

Disposition: The patient tolerated the procedure well, and there were no apparent complications. Vital signs remained stable throughout the procedure. The patient was taken to the recovery area where written discharge instructions for the procedure were given. **[POSTOP PLAN IS ...]**

Subacromial Bursa Injection

Patient Name: MR#: Date of Procedure:
Preoperative Diagnosis: **[Shoulder Pain; Impingement Syndrome]**
Postoperative Diagnosis: **[Shoulder Pain; Impingement Syndrome]**

Operation Title:
1) **[Right/Left]** Subacromial Bursa Injection

Attending Physician:
Assistant Physician:

Indications: The patient is a **[age]** old **[male/female]** with a diagnosis of **[Right/Left]** **[shoulder pain; impingement syndrome]**. This is the **[x]** injection of **[#]**. **[The patient had [X]% relief from the previous injection.]** The patient's history and physical exam have been reviewed. The risks, benefits, and alternatives to the procedure have been discussed, and all questions have been answered to the patient's satisfaction. The patient agreed to proceed and written informed consent was obtained.

Procedure in Detail: The patient was brought into the procedure room and placed in the **[sitting]** position on the fluoroscopy table. The **[right/left]** upper extremity was placed to the patient's side. The shoulder was then prepped with chloroprep times 3 and draped in a sterile manner. The acromion was then palpated anteriorly and laterally until the antero-lateral corner was located. The skin and subcutaneous tissues in the area were anesthetized with ethyl chloride spray. With an index finger on the lateral acromion, a **[25-gauge 3.5 inch]** needle was inserted about 1 cm below the palpating finger and advanced while angled superiorly 20–30 degrees to access the subacromial space. There was no resistance to needle entry. After negative aspiration, a solution containing **[2 mL 1% lidocaine, 2 mL 0.25% bupivacaine and 40 mg triamcinolone]** was administered. The needle was then withdrawn with a saline flush. The shoulder was cleaned and a bandage was placed over the site of needle insertion. Active and passive full range of motion was then tested to promote distribution of the steroid.

Disposition: The patient tolerated the procedure well, and there were no apparent complications. Vital signs remained stable throughout the procedure. The patient was taken to the recovery area where written discharge instructions for the procedure were given. **[POSTOP PLAN IS ...]**

Glenohumeral Intra-Articular Injection

Patient Name: MR#: Date of Procedure:
Preoperative Diagnosis: **[Glenohumeral joint Osteoarthritis]**
Postoperative Diagnosis: **[Glenohumeral joint Osteoarthritis]**

Operation Title:
1) **[Right/Left]** Intra-Articular Shoulder Injection

Attending Physician:
Assistant Physician:
Anesthesia: Local

Indications: The patient is a **[age]** old **[male/female]** with a diagnosis of **[Right/Left] [Glenohumeral joint Osteoarthritis and Shoulder pain]**. This is the **[x]** injection of **[#]**. **[The patient had [X]% relief from the previous injection.]** The patient's history and physical exam have been reviewed. The risks, benefits, and alternatives to the procedure have been discussed, and all questions have been answered to the patient's satisfaction. The patient agreed to proceed and written informed consent was obtained.

Procedure in Detail: The patient was placed in a seated position with **[right/left]** shoulder internally rotated. A point of needle insertion was marked approximately 2 cm inferior and medial to the posterior lateral edge of the acromion. The area of the **[right/left]** posterior shoulder was prepped with ChloraPrep times three. The skin and subcutaneous tissues in this area were anesthetized with 1% lidocaine. A 25-gauge 1.5 inch needle was directed anterior medially toward the coracoid process. After negative aspiration was confirmed, a solution consisting of **[1 mL of 40 mg depomedrol]** and **[4 mL] [1% lidocaine]** was easily injected. The needle was removed. The patient's posterior shoulder was cleaned and a bandage was placed over the site of needle insertion.

Disposition: The patient tolerated the procedure well, and there were no apparent complications. Vital signs remained stable throughout the procedure. The patient was taken to the recovery area where written discharge instructions for the procedure were given. **[POSTOP PLAN IS ...]**

Acromioclavicular Joint Injection

Patient Name: MR#: Date **[AC joint Osteoarthritis]**
Postoperative Diagnosis: **[AC joint Osteoarthritis]**

Operation Title:
1) **[Right/Left]** AC Joint Injection

Attending Physician:
Assistant Physician:
Anesthesia: Local

Indications: The patient is a **[age]** old **[male/female]** with a diagnosis of **[Right/Left] [AC joint Osteoarthritis and Shoulder pain]**. This is the **[x]** injection of **[#]**. **[The patient had [X]% relief from the previous injection.]** The patient's history and physical exam have been reviewed. The risks, benefits, and alternatives to the procedure have been discussed, and all questions have been answered to the patient's satisfaction. The patient agreed to proceed and written informed consent was obtained.

Procedure in Detail: The patient was placed in a seated position with **[right/left]** shoulder resting at side. After identifying the acromion and clavicle, a point of needle insertion was marked at the superior/anterior AC joint. The area of the **[right/left]** AC joint was prepped with ChloraPrep times 3. The skin and subcutaneous tissues in this area were anesthetized with 1% lidocaine. A 25-gauge 1.5 inch needle was inserted from a superior/anterior approach and directed inferiorly toward the AC joint until capsule was entered. After negative aspiration was confirmed, a solution consisting of **[1 mL of 40 mg depomedrol]** and **[1 mL] [1% lidocaine]** was easily injected. The needle was removed. The patient's anterior shoulder was cleaned and a bandage was placed over the site of needle insertion.

Disposition: The patient tolerated the procedure well, and there were no apparent complications. Vital signs remained stable throughout the procedure. The patient was taken to the recovery area where written discharge instructions for the procedure were given. **[POSTOP PLAN IS ...]**

Trigger Finger Injection

Patient Name: MR#: Date of Procedure:
Preoperative Diagnosis: **[Right/Left Trigger Finger]**
Postoperative Diagnosis: **[Right/Left Trigger Finger]**

Operation Title:
1) **[Right/Left]** Trigger Finger Injection

Attending Physician:
Assistant Physician:

Indications: The patient is a **[age]** old **[male/female]** with a diagnosis of **[Right/Left]** **[Trigger Finger]**. This is the **[x]** injection of **[#]**. **[The patient had [X]% relief from the previous injection.]** The patient's history and physical exam have been reviewed. The risks, benefits, and alternatives to the procedure have been discussed, and all questions have been answered to the patient's satisfaction. The patient agreed to proceed and written informed consent was obtained.

Procedure in Detail:
The patient was placed in a **[sitting/supine]** position. The patient assisted in localizing the point of maximal tenderness in her **[right/left finger]**. The palpable nodules on the **[right/left finger]** flexor tendons were identified at the metacarpophalangeal joint. The point of maximal tenderness was palpated and location of the sliding of the tendon nodule through the retinaculum was also identified and marked. These areas were then cleansed with ChloraPrep. **[The skin was numbed using topical ethyl chloride.]** The skin was then again recleansed using ChloraPrep. A **[27-gauge1.25 inch]** needle was attached to a 5 mL syringe filled with **[40 mg of Kenalog and 2 mL of 1% lidocaine for a total volume of 3 mL]**. The needle was inserted just lateral to tendon nodule. The needle was advanced into the tendon sheath as the patient moved the affected finger through a small arc of flexion and extension. When the needle touched the moving tendon, the patient experienced a gritty sensation and needle advancement stopped. The needle was then withdrawn until there was no motion felt in the needle with a movement of the patient's finger. At this point, an injection of **[1.5 mL of the combination of Kenalog and 1% lidocaine was performed]** at the site after negative aspiration. The needle was then removed. The patient's hand was then cleansed and bands placed over the site of needle insertion. **[The procedure was repeated on the _____ finger.]**

Disposition: The patient tolerated the procedure well, and there were no apparent complications. Vital signs remained stable throughout the procedure. The patient was taken to the recovery area where written discharge instructions for the procedure were given. **[POSTOP PLAN IS ...]**

Stellate Ganglion Block

Patient Name: MR#: Date of Procedure:
Preoperative Diagnosis: **[CRPS of the right/left arm/other]**
Postoperative Diagnosis: **[CRPS of the right/left arm/other]**

Operation Title:
1) **[right/left]** Stellate Ganglion Block; 2) Intraoperative Fluoroscopy;
3) **[IV Conscious Sedation]**

Attending Physician:
Assistant Physician:
Anesthesia: Local **[and conscious sedation with ...]**

Indications: The patient is a **[age]** old **[male/female]** with a diagnosis of **[diagnosis]**. This is the **[x]** injection of **[#]**. **[The patient had [X]% relief from the previous injection.]** The patient's history and physical exam have been reviewed. The risks, benefits, and alternatives to the procedure have been discussed, and all questions have been answered to the patient's satisfaction. The patient agreed to proceed and written informed consent was obtained.

Procedure in Detail: [An IV was started while the patient was in the preoperative holding area.] The patient was brought into the procedure room and placed in the supine position on the fluoroscopy table with the head turned to the **[right/left]** side. Neck extension was obtained by placing a towel underneath the shoulders. Standard monitors were placed, and vital signs were observed throughout the procedure. The area of the neck was prepped with chloroprep times three and draped in a sterile manner. AP fluoroscopy with caudal tilt was used to identify the **[right/left]** C7 transverse process and the intravertebral disk spaces were aligned. Then, the fluoroscopic beam was obliqued to the **[left/right]** side to visualize the junction of the uncinate process and the vertebral body of C7. This area was then marked. The site of entry was then anesthetized with 1% lidocaine and the skin wheal was raised at the surface point. Under fluoroscopic guidance, a single pass was made with a **[25-gauge 3-1/2 inch]** needle to contact the bone with caution to avoid passage of the needle toward the neuroforamina posteriorly and the disk located in the anterior. The needle tip was then placed at the junction of the uncinate process and the vertebral body. Next, 1 mL of radiopaque dye was injected with imaging including digital subtraction imaging confirming distribution around the stellate ganglion and avoiding intravascular spread.

Stellate Ganglion Block *(Continued)*

Then, a test dose of 0.5 mL of 0.25% bupivacaine was injected. The patient was observed for any symptoms of ringing in the ears, metallic taste in the mouth, dizziness, or perioral numbness for 30 seconds. This was negative. Then, a solution containing 10 mg of dexamethasone and 4 mL of 0.25% bupivacaine, total volume of 5 mL was injected under intermittent negative aspiration and under fluoroscopic guidance. The patient confirmed with hand signals that **[he/she]** was tolerating the procedure well. The needle was then removed, the patient's back was cleaned and a bandage was placed over the site of needle insertion.

Disposition: The patient tolerated the procedure well, and there were no apparent complications. Vital signs remained stable throughout the procedure. The patient was taken to the recovery area where written discharge instructions for the procedure were given. **[POSTOP PLAN IS ...]**

Ganglion Impar Block

Patient Name: MR#: Date of Procedure:
Preoperative Diagnosis: **[Coccygodynia; Pelvic Pain]**
Postoperative Diagnosis: **[Coccygodynia; Pelvic Pain]**

Operation Title:
1) Ganglion Impar Block; 2) Intraoperative Fluoroscopy; 3) **[IV Conscious Sedation]**

Attending Physician:
Assistant Physician:
Anesthesia: Local **[and conscious sedation with ...]**

Indications: The patient is a **[age]** old **[male/female]** with a diagnosis of **[coccygodynia; pelvic pain]**. This is the **[x]** injection of **[#]**. **[The patient had [X]% relief from the previous injection.]** The patient's history and physical exam have been reviewed. The risks, benefits, and alternatives to the procedure have been discussed, and all questions have been answered to the patient's satisfaction. The patient agreed to proceed and written informed consent was obtained.

Procedure in Detail: [An IV was started while the patient was in the pre-operative holding area.] The patient was brought into the procedure room and placed in the prone position on the fluoroscopy table. Standard monitors were placed, and vital signs were observed throughout the procedure. The area of the sacrococcygeal junction was visualized under lateral fluoroscopy; the skin was then prepped with chloroprep times three and draped in a sterile manner. The skin and subcutaneous tissues in the area were anesthetized with 1% lidocaine. A **[22-gauge 3.5 inch]** needle was placed through the sacrococcygeal ligament. In the lateral view, the needle was advanced under fluoroscopic guidance until the tip was just anterior to the sacrococcygeal ligament. Negative aspiration was confirmed and 1 mL of contrast solution was injected. A vertical concave contrast spread along the anterior sacrococcygeal junction was observed, consistent with the "comma sign." After negative aspiration, a solution consisting of **[80 mg triamcinolone]** and **[4 mL]** preservative-free saline was easily injected. The needle was removed with a saline flush. The patient's back was cleaned and a bandage was placed over the site of needle insertion.

Disposition: The patient tolerated the procedure well, and there were no apparent complications. Vital signs remained stable throughout the procedure. The patient was taken to the recovery area where written discharge instructions for the procedure were given. **[POSTOP PLAN IS ...]**

Lumbar Sympathetic Block

Patient Name: MR#: Date of Procedure:
Preoperative Diagnosis: **[CRPS of the right/left leg; Other diagnosis]**
Postoperative Diagnosis: **[CRPS of the right/left leg; Other diagnosis]**

Operation Title:
1) **[[Right/left] XX]** Lumbar Sympathetic Block; 2) Intraoperative
Fluoroscopy; 3) **[IV Conscious Sedation]**

Attending Physician:
Assistant Physician:
Anesthesia: Local **[and conscious sedation with ...]**

Indications: The patient is a **[age]** old **[male/female]** with a diagnosis
of **[diagnosis]**. This is the **[x]** injection of **[#]**. **[The patient had [X]%
relief from the previous injection.]** The patient's history and physical
exam have been reviewed. The risks, benefits, and alternatives to the
procedure have been discussed, and all questions have been answered
to the patient's satisfaction. The patient agreed to proceed and written
informed consent was obtained.

**Procedure in Detail: [An IV was started while the patient was in the
preoperative holding area.]** The patient was brought into the procedure room and placed in the prone position on the fluoroscopy table.
Standard monitors were placed, and vital signs were observed throughout the procedure. The area of the lumbar spine was prepped with chloroprep times three and draped in a sterile manner. The **[XX]** vertebral
body was identified and marked under AP fluoroscopy. An oblique view
to the **[right/left]** was obtained such that the lateral aspect of the **[XX]**
transverse process on the **[right/left]** was overlying the lateral margin of
the vertebral body. A target point was chosen at the inferior margin of
the transverse process, adjacent to the vertebral body. The skin and subcutaneous tissues were anesthetized with 1% lidocaine using a 25-gauge
1.5 inch needle followed by a 22-gauge 3.5 inch needle. A 22-gauge
6.5 inch needle was then directed under intermittent fluoroscopy and
advanced parallel to the fluoroscopic beam. The needle tip was slowly
walked off inferiorly below the transverse process. **[The same procedure was repeated at the [XX] level.]** Lateral fluoroscopy was then used
to advance the needle tip to the anterior margin of the vertebral body.
After negative aspiration was confirmed, 1 mL of contrast was injected
at each level, showing good spread along the distribution of the lumbar
sympathetic chain on both lateral and AP fluoroscopy. Then, after reconfirming negative aspiration, 10 mL of 0.25% bupivacaine was injected
at each level. The needle(s) were then removed. The patient's back was
cleaned and bandages were placed over the sites of needle insertion.

Lumbar Sympathetic Block (*Continued*)

Disposition: The patient tolerated the procedure well, and there were no apparent complications. Vital signs remained stable throughout the procedure. The patient was taken to the recovery area where written discharge instructions for the procedure were given. **[POSTOP PLAN IS ...]**

Postop Exam and Temperature Changes: [XXXXXXXX]

Celiac Plexus Block

Patient Name: MR#: Date of Procedure:
Preoperative Diagnosis: **[diagnosis]**
Postoperative Diagnosis: **[diagnosis]**

Operation Title:
1) **[Right/ Left]** Celiac Plexus Block; 2) Intraoperative Fluoroscopy;
3) **[IV Conscious Sedation]**

Attending Physician:
Assistant Physician:
Anesthesia: Local **[and conscious sedation with ...]**

Indications: The patient is a **[age]** old **[male/female]** with a diagnosis of **[diagnosis]**. This is the **[x]** injection of **[#]**. **[The patient had [X]% relief from the previous injection.]** The patient's history and physical exam have been reviewed. The risks, benefits, and alternatives to the procedure have been discussed, and all questions have been answered to the patient's satisfaction. The patient agreed to proceed and written informed consent was obtained.

Procedure in Detail: [An IV was started while the patient was in the preoperative holding area.] The patient was brought into the procedure room and placed in the prone position on the fluoroscopy table. Standard monitors were placed, and vital signs were observed throughout the procedure. The area of the thoracolumbar spine was prepped with chloroprep times three and draped in a sterile manner. The **[L1]** vertebral body was identified and marked under AP fluoroscopy. A **[7/7.5/8 cm]** point on the **[right/left]** was measured laterally from the spinous process and marked. A far oblique view to the **[right/left]** was then obtained until the marked point was seen to overlap the lateral border of the vertebral body. This point was then remarked just slightly inferior to the transverse process. The twelfth rib was visualized to lie lateral to the marked point. The skin and subcutaneous tissues in the area were then anesthetized with 1% lidocaine. A 22-gauge **[5 inch]** needle was then directed under intermittent fluoroscopy and advanced parallel to the fluoroscopic beam until the lateral border of the vertebral body was contacted. The needle was then walked off the vertebral body laterally. Lateral fluoroscopy was then used to advance the needle tip to the anterior margin of the vertebral body. After negative aspiration was confirmed, 1 mL of contrast was injected, showing good spread along the distribution of the plexus on both lateral and AP fluoroscopy.

Celiac Plexus Block (*Continued*)

Then, after reconfirming negative aspiration, **[10 mL]** of **[0.25% bupi-vacaine]** was injected, with intermittent aspiration and pauses every 2–3 mL to reconfirm lack of vascular uptake.

[The same procedure was then repeated on the contralateral side.]

The needle(s) were then removed. The patient's back was cleaned and bandages were placed over the sites of needle insertion.

Disposition: The patient tolerated the procedure well, and there were no apparent complications. Vital signs remained stable throughout the procedure. The patient was taken to the recovery area where written discharge instructions for the procedure were given. **[POSTOP PLAN IS ...]**

Ilioinguinal/Iliohypogastric Block

Patient Name: MR#: Date of Procedure:
Preoperative Diagnosis: **[Ilioinguinal/Iliohypogastric Neuralgia]**
Postoperative Diagnosis: **[Ilioinguinal/Iliohypogastric Neuralgia]**

Operation Title:
1) Ilioinguinal/Iliohypogastric Nerve Block; 2) Intraoperative
Fluoroscopy; 3) **[IV Conscious Sedation]**

Attending Physician:
Assistant Physician:
Anesthesia: Local **[and conscious sedation with ...]**

Indications: The patient is a **[age]** old **[male/female]** with a diagnosis of
[Ilioinguinal/Iliohypogastric neuralgia]. This is the **[x]** injection of **[#]**.
[The patient had [X]% relief from the previous injection.] The patient's
history and physical exam have been reviewed. The risks, benefits, and
alternatives to the procedure have been discussed, and all questions
have been answered to the patient's satisfaction. The patient agreed to
proceed and written informed consent was obtained.

**Procedure in Detail: [An IV was started while the patient was in the
pre-operative holding area.]** The patient was brought into the procedure room and placed in the supine position on the fluoroscopy table.
Standard monitors were placed, and vital signs were observed throughout the procedure. The groin and inguinal area were prepped with chloroprep times three and draped in a sterile manner. The anterior superior
iliac spine was identified and marked under AP fluoroscopy. **[A point 2
cm medial and caudal was marked for the Ilioinguinal Nerve.] [A point
1 cm medial and caudal was marked for the Iliohypogastric Nerve.]** The
skin and subcutaneous tissues in the area were anesthetized with 1%
lidocaine. A **[22-gauge 3.5 inch]** needle was inserted until two separate
pops were felt indicating passage through two fascial planes. The needle
therefore lies between the internal and external oblique muscles.

Negative aspiration was confirmed and 1 mL of contrast solution was
injected. After negative aspiration, a solution consisting of **[80 mg
triamcinolone]** and **[4 mL]** preservative-free saline was easily injected.
The needle was removed with a saline flush. The patient's back was
cleaned and a bandage was placed over the site of needle insertion.

Disposition: The patient tolerated the procedure well, and there were
no apparent complications. Vital signs remained stable throughout the
procedure. The patient was taken to the recovery area where written discharge instructions for the procedure were given. **[POSTOP PLAN IS ...]**

Pudendal Nerve Block

Patient Name: MR#: Date of Procedure:
Preoperative Diagnosis: **[Pudendal Neuralgia]**
Postoperative Diagnosis: **[Pudendal Neuralgia]**

Operation Title:
1) **[Right/left]** Pudendal Nerve Block; 2) Intraoperative Fluoroscopy;
3) **[IV Conscious Sedation]**

Attending Physician:
Assistant Physician:
Anesthesia: Local **[and conscious sedation with ...]**

Indications: The patient is a **[age]** old **[male/female]** with a diagnosis of **[Pudendal neuralgia]**. This is the **[x]** injection of **[#]**. **[The patient had [X]% relief from the previous injection.]** The patient's history and physical exam have been reviewed. The risks, benefits, and alternatives to the procedure have been discussed, and all questions have been answered to the patient's satisfaction. The patient agreed to proceed and written informed consent was obtained.

Procedure in Detail: [An IV was started while the patient was in the pre-operative holding area.] The patient was brought into the procedure room and placed in the prone position on the fluoroscopy table. Standard monitors were placed, and vital signs were observed throughout the procedure. The **[right/left]** buttock area was prepped with chloroprep times three and draped in a sterile manner. The ischial spine was identified under AP fluoroscopy with a slight caudal and slight oblique tilt. The skin and subcutaneous tissues in the area were anesthetized with 1% lidocaine. A **[22-gauge 3.5 inch]** needle was advanced toward the ischial spine under fluoroscopic guidance until bone was contacted. The needle was then walked off bone in a **[supero/infero]** medial fashion. Then after negative aspiration, a solution consisting of **[80 mg triamcinolone and 2 mL 0.25% bupivacaine]** was easily injected. The needle was then removed with a saline flush. The patient's back was cleaned and a bandage was placed over the site of needle insertion.

Disposition: The patient tolerated the procedure well, and there were no apparent complications. Vital signs remained stable throughout the procedure. The patient was taken to the recovery area where written discharge instructions for the procedure were given. **[POSTOP PLAN IS ...]**

Discography

Patient Name: MR#: Date of Procedure:
Preoperative Diagnosis: **[Cervical/Thoracic/Lumbar Degenerative Disc Disease]**
Postoperative Diagnosis: **[Cerv/Th/Lumbar Deg. Disc Disease]**

Operation Title:
1) **[XX-XX]** Discography; 2) Intraoperative Fluoroscopy; 3) **[IV Conscious Sedation]**

Attending Physician:
Assistant Physician:
Anesthesia: Local **[and conscious sedation with ...]**

Indications: The patient is a **[age]** old **[male/female]** with a diagnosis of **[degenerative disc disease]**. The patient is here today for a diagnostic discography. The patient's history and physical exam have been reviewed. The risks, benefits, and alternatives to the procedure have been discussed, and all questions have been answered to the patient's satisfaction. The patient agreed to proceed and written informed consent was obtained.

Procedure in Detail: [An IV was started while the patient was in the preoperative holding area.] The patient received an intravenous infusion of **[XX mg abx]** over a half hour. The patient was brought into the procedure room and placed in the prone position on the fluoroscopy table. Standard monitors were placed, and vital signs were observed throughout the procedure. The area of the **[cervical/thoracic/lumbar]** spine was prepped with chloroprep times three and draped in a sterile manner. The **[XX-XX]** disc space was identified and marked under AP fluoroscopy. An oblique view to the **[right]** was obtained to overlap the facet joint over the midpoint of the disc space. A target point was then chosen just lateral to the facet joint. The skin and subcutaneous tissues in the area were anesthetized with 1% lidocaine. A 22-gauge 6.5 inch needle was directed toward the targeted point under fluoroscopy until the disc was entered. Discs at the other specified levels were entered in a similar fashion.

AP and cross table fluoroscopy were used to properly place the needle tip in the center of the disc. Once all the needles were in proper position, disc provocation was done with the following results:

Disc: **[XX-XX]**; Volume: **[XX mL]**; Consistency: **[firm/free-flowing]**; Morphology: **[normal/degenerative]**; Pain: **[none/concordant/non-concordant]**

1 mL of 0.25% bupivacaine was then injected to anesthetize each disc. All needles were removed. The patient's back was cleaned and bandages were placed over the sites of needle insertion.

Discography (*Continued*)

Disposition: The patient tolerated the procedure well, and there were no apparent complications. Vital signs remained stable throughout the procedure. The patient was taken to the recovery area where written discharge instructions for the procedure were given. The patient was given a prescription for **[abx prophylaxis for 3–5 days; state sig and # dispensed]**.

[POSTOP PLAN IS ...]

DISCHARGE ANTIBIOTICS When appropriate

Keflex 500 mg qid × 10 days

For Penicillin Allergy:
Clindamycin 300 mg q6 hr × 10 days

Radiofrequency Ablation (RFA): Cervical Medial Branch

Patient Name: MR#: Date of Procedure:
Preoperative Diagnosis: **[Cervical Facet Arthropathy]**
Postoperative Diagnosis: **[Cervical Facet Arthropathy]**

Operation Title:
1) Radiofrequency Ablation of the **[Right/left/bilateral XX-XX]** medial branch nerves; 2) Intraoperative Fluoroscopy; 3) **[IV Conscious Sedation]**

Attending Physician:
Assistant Physician:
Anesthesia: Local **[and conscious sedation with ...]**

Indications: The patient is a **[age]** old **[male/female]** with a diagnosis of **[cervical facet arthropathy]**. The patient's history and physical exam have been reviewed. The risks, benefits, and alternatives to the procedure have been discussed, and all questions have been answered to the patient's satisfaction. The patient agreed to proceed and written informed consent was obtained.

Procedure in Detail: The patient was brought into the procedure room and placed in the prone position on the fluoroscopy table. Standard monitors were placed and vital signs were observed throughout the procedure. The area of the cervical spine was prepped with chloroprep times three and draped in a sterile manner. AP fluoroscopy with a 25–35 degree caudal tilt was used to visualize the articular pillars. The midpoint between the superior and inferior articular processes of each targeted facet is marked; this point appeared as an invagination where the lateral margin of the facet column dips medially between the articular surfaces. These points were marked at the **[XX-XX]** levels on the **[right/left]** side. The skin and subcutaneous tissues in these identified areas were anesthetized with 1% lidocaine. A 10 cm SMK cannulae with 5 mm active tip is advanced toward each of these points under fluoroscopic guidance. Once bone was contacted, the needle was walked off the facet column laterally and advanced 2–3 mm to position the active tip along the course of the medial branch nerve. Negative aspiration was confirmed. Sensory stimulation was performed at 50 Hz and 0.4 V, generating a pressure sensation. Motor stimulation at 2 Hz and 1.2 V was negative. **[0.5 mL]** of **[2% lidocaine]** was injected at each level prior to lesioning, which was performed for **[90 seconds at 80 degrees]** Centigrade. Once the lesion was complete, 0.5 mL of a solution consisting of 4 mL 0.25% bupivacaine and 40 mg triamcinolone was injected through each probe. The probes were removed with a 1% lidocaine flush.

[The same procedure was repeated on the opposite side.]

Radiofrequency Ablation (RFA): Cervical Medial Branch
(Continued)

After the procedure was completed, the patient's neck was cleaned and bandages were placed at the needle insertion sites.

Disposition: The patient tolerated the procedure well and there were no apparent complications. Vital signs remained stable throughout the procedure. The patient was taken to the recovery area where written discharge instructions for the procedure were given. **[POSTOP PLAN IS ...]**

RFA: Lumbar Medial Branch

Patient Name: MR#: Date of Procedure:
Preoperative Diagnosis: **[Lumbar Facet Arthropathy]**
Postoperative Diagnosis: **[Lumbar Facet Arthropathy]**

Operation Title:
1) Radiofrequency Ablation of the **[Right/left/bilateral XX-XX]** medial branch nerves; 2) Intraoperative Fluoroscopy; 3) **[IV Conscious Sedation]**

Attending Physician:
Assistant Physician:
Anesthesia: Local **[and conscious sedation with ...]**

Indications: The patient is a **[age]** old **[male/female]** with a diagnosis of **[lumbar facet arthropathy]**. The patient's history and physical exam were reviewed. The risks, benefits, and alternatives to the procedure have been discussed; all questions were answered to the patient's satisfaction. The patient agreed to proceed and written informed consent was obtained.

Procedure in Detail: [An IV was started while the patient was in the preoperative holding area.] The patient was brought into the procedure room and placed in the prone position on the fluoroscopy table. Standard monitors were placed and vital signs were observed throughout the procedure. The area of the lumbar spine was prepped with chloroprep times three and draped in a sterile manner. AP and oblique fluoroscopy were used to identify and mark the junctions between the superior articular processes and transverse processes at the **[XX-XX]** levels on the **[right/left]** side. **[The sacral ala and the 2 o'clock/10 o'clock position of the right/left S1 foramen were identified and marked.]** The skin and subcutaneous tissues in these identified areas were anesthetized with 1% lidocaine. A 22-gauge 100 mm probe radiofrequency probe was advanced toward each of these points under fluoroscopic guidance. Once bone was contacted, negative aspiration was confirmed. Sensory stimulation was performed at 50 Hz and 0.4 V, generating a pressure sensation. Motor stimulation at 2 Hz and 1.2 V was negative. **[1 mL]** of **[2% lidocaine]** was injected at each level prior to lesioning, which was performed for **[90 seconds at 90 degrees]** Centigrade. Once the lesion was complete, 1 mL of a solution consisting of 4 mL 0.25% bupivacaine and 40 mg triamcinolone was injected through each probe. The probes were removed with a 1% lidocaine flush. **[The same procedure was repeated on the opposite side.]**

After the procedure was completed, the patient's back was cleaned and bandages were placed at the needle insertion sites.

Disposition: The patient tolerated the procedure well and there were no apparent complications. Vital signs remained stable throughout the procedure. The patient was taken to the recovery area where written discharge instructions for the procedure were given. **[POSTOP PLAN IS ...]**

RFA: Strip Lesioning Sacroiliac (SI) Joint

Patient Name: MR#: Date of Procedure:
Preoperative Diagnosis: **[Sacroiliac Dysfunction]**
Postoperative Diagnosis: **[Sacroiliac Dysfunction]**

Operation Title:
1) Radiofrequency Strip Lesioning of the **[Right/left]** Sacroiliac Joint;
2) Intraoperative Fluoroscopy; 3) **[IV Conscious Sedation]**

Attending Physician:
Assistant Physician:
Anesthesia: Local **[and conscious sedation with ...]**

Indications: The patient is a **[age]** old **[male/female]** with a diagnosis of **[sacroiliac dysfunction]**. The patient's history and physical exam were reviewed. The risks, benefits, and alternatives to the procedure have been discussed; all questions were answered to the patient's satisfaction. The patient agreed to proceed and written informed consent was obtained.

Procedure in Detail: [An IV was started while the patient was in the pre-operative holding area.] The patient was brought into the procedure room and placed in the prone position on the fluoroscopy table. Standard monitors were placed and vital signs were observed throughout the procedure. The area of the lumbar spine and upper buttock were prepped with chloroprep times three and draped in a sterile manner. AP fluoroscopy was used to visualize the **[right/left]** sacroiliac joint. The fluoroscopic beam was then oblique until the anterior and posterior margins of the joint were aligned. The inferior margin of the joint was identified and marked. The skin and subcutaneous tissues in the area were anesthetized with 1% lidocaine. A 22-gauge 100 mm radiofrequency probe was advanced toward the identified point under fluoroscopic guidance. Once the targeted point was reached and the joint space was entered, negative aspiration was confirmed and 1 mL of contrast was injected. The joint space was appropriately outlined. Then, after negative aspiration, a solution containing **[X mL of 0.25% bupivacaine and XX mg of triamcinolone]** was easily injected. A second probe was placed approximately 1 cm above the first needle in the joint space. A bipolar lesion was performed for 90 seconds at 90 degrees Centigrade. This procedure was repeated in the joint until **[X]** lesions were completed. All needles were removed with a 1% lidocaine flush. The patient's back was cleaned and bandages were placed at the needle insertion sites.

Disposition: The patient tolerated the procedure well and there were no apparent complications. Vital signs remained stable throughout the procedure. The patient was taken to the recovery area where written discharge instructions for the procedure were given. **[POSTOP PLAN IS ...]**

RFA: Denervation of SI Joint

Patient Name: MR#: Date of Procedure:
Preoperative Diagnosis: **[Sacroiliac Dysfunction]**
Postoperative Diagnosis: **[Sacroiliac Dysfunction]**

Operation Title:
1) Radiofrequency Ablation of the **[Right/Left]** L4 and L5 dorsal rami
2) Radiofrequency Ablation of the **[Right/Left]** S1-S3 Lateral Branch Nerves
3) Intraoperative Fluoroscopy
4) **[IV Conscious Sedation]**

Attending Physician:
Assistant Physician:
Anesthesia: Local **[and conscious sedation with ...]**

Indications: This is a **[age]** old **[male/female]** with a diagnosis of **[sacroiliac dysfunction]**. The patient's history and physical exam have been reviewed. The risks, benefits, and alternatives to the procedure have been discussed, and all questions have been answered to the patient's satisfaction. The patient agreed to proceed and a written informed consent was obtained.

Procedure in Detail: [An IV was started while the patient was in the preoperative holding area.] The patient was brought into the procedure room and placed in the prone position on the fluoroscopy table. Standard monitors were placed, and vital signs were observed throughout the procedure. The areas of the low back and upper buttock were prepped with chloroprep times three and draped in a sterile manner. AP fluoroscopy was used to identify and mark the junction between the superior border of the transverse process and superior articular process for the L4 dorsal rami on the **[right/left]** side. AP fluoroscopy was used to identify and mark the junction of the sacral ala and the articular process of the sacrum for the L5 dorsal rami on the **[right/left]** side. The skin and subcutaneous tissues in these identified areas were anesthetized with 1% lidocaine. A **[22-gauge 100 mm radiofrequency probe]** was advanced toward each of these points under fluoroscopic guidance. Sensory stimulation was performed at 50 Hz and 0.4 V, generating a pressure sensation. Motor stimulation at 2 Hz and 1.2 V was negative. **[0.5 mL]** of **[2% lidocaine]** was injected at each level prior to lesioning, which was performed for **[90 seconds at 80 degrees]** Centigrade. AP fluoroscopy was then used to mark and identify the S1–S3 lateral branches at approximately 3–5 mm from the lateral foramina of the respective foramen. **[The right-sided S1 and S2 lateral branch nerves correspond to approximately the 1:00, 3:00, and 5:30 positions.] [The left-sided S1 and S2 lateral branch nerves correspond to approximately the 6:30, 9:00, and 11:00 positions.] [The right-sided S3 lateral branch nerves correspond to the 1:30 and 4:30 positions].**

RFA: Denervation of SI Joint (*Continued*)

[The left-sided S3 lateral branch nerves correspond to the 7:30 and 10:30 positions.] [17-gauge, 75-mm cooled electrodes] were inserted into each of these points under fluoroscopic guidance. Sensory stimulation was performed at 50 Hz and 0.4 V, generating a pressure sensation. [0.5 mL] of [2% lidocaine] was injected at each level. Monopolar electrodes were then inserted into the cannulae, and 2.5-min lesions were made using a watercooled radiofrequency heating system, keeping the tissue temperature immediately adjacent to the cooled electrode at 60°C, while the target tissue at 75°C. [The same procedure was repeated on the opposite side.] After the procedure was completed, the patient's back was cleaned and bandages were placed at the needle insertion sites.

Disposition: The patient tolerated the procedure well and there were no apparent complications. Vital signs remained stable throughout the procedure. The patient was taken to the recovery area where written discharge instructions for the procedure were given. [POSTOP PLAN IS ...]

Spinal Cord Stimulator Trial

Patient Name: MR#: Date of Procedure:
Preoperative Diagnosis: **[diagnosis]**
Postoperative Diagnosis: **[diagnosis]**

Operation Title:
1) Percutaneous placement of trial spinal cord stimulator leads times **[Number]**; 2) Intraoperative Fluoroscopy; 3) **[IV Conscious Sedation]**

Attending Physician:
Assistant Physician:
Anesthesia: Local **[and conscious sedation with ...]**

Indications: The patient is a **[age]** old **[male/female]** with a diagnosis of **[diagnosis]**. The patient's history and physical exam were reviewed. The risks, benefits, and alternatives to the procedure have been discussed; all questions were answered to the patient's satisfaction. The patient agreed to proceed and written informed consent was obtained.

Procedure in Detail: [An IV was started while the patient was in the preoperative holding area.] The patient was brought into the procedure room and placed in the prone position on the fluoroscopy table. An intravenous infusion of **[Abx]** was started and completed over one hour. Standard monitors were placed and vital signs were observed throughout the procedure. The area of the **[cervical/thoracic/lumbar]** spine was prepped with alcohol times three, then Hibiclens times three, then ChloraPrep scrub times three then betadine paint times three and draped in a sterile manner. The surgical site was covered with an Ioban covering.

The **[XX-XX]** interspace was identified. The skin and subcutaneous tissues in the area were anesthetized with 1% lidocaine. A 14-gauge Tuohy epidural needle was advanced with a paramedian approach from the **[right/left]** using a loss of resistance technique with a glass syringe and air in order to identify entrance into the epidural space. Once a good loss of resistance was obtained, negative aspiration was confirmed. An **[8]** contact lead was advanced under fluoroscopic guidance until the 0-position was at **[upper/mid/lower XX vertebral body level]. [A second lead was placed using the same technique from the XX-XX interspace on the right/left until the 0-position was at the upper/mid/lower XX vertebral body level.]** The leads were connected to an external trial programmer using sterile connectors. Several combinations of lead configuration, frequency, amplitude, and pulse width were used until comfortable, appropriate coverage of the patient's pain area was obtained.

Spinal Cord Stimulator Trial (*Continued*)

The needle(s) were then carefully removed and the lead(s) were secured to the skin using **[chest tube type ties]** and 2-0 silk suture. Fluoroscopy was used to confirm continued proper placement of the lead(s) before being anchored. The skin was covered with **[antibiotic ointment and covered with a gauze dressing]**. The connectors were also wrapped in gauze and secured to the patient.

Disposition: The patient tolerated the procedure well and there were no apparent complications. Vital signs remained stable throughout the procedure. The patient was taken to the recovery area where written discharge instructions for the procedure were given. **[POSTOP PLAN IS ...]**

SCS Implantation

Patient Name: MR#: Date of Procedure:
Preoperative Diagnosis: **[diagnosis]**
Postoperative Diagnosis: **[diagnosis]**

Operation Title:
1) Implantation of permanent spinal cord stimulator leads × **[Number]**;
2) Implantation of IPG Unit; 3) Intraoperative Fluoroscopy

Attending Physician:
Assistant Physician:
Anesthesia: Monitored anesthesia care

Indications: The patient is a **[age]** old **[male/female]** with a diagnosis of **[diagnosis]**. **[He/she]** is here today for permanent implantation of spinal cord stimulator lead(s) and an IPG unit. The patient's history and physical exam were reviewed. The risks, benefits, and alternatives to the procedure have been discussed; all questions were answered to the patient's satisfaction. The patient agreed to proceed and written informed consent was obtained.

Procedure in Detail: [An IV was started while the patient was in the preoperative holding area.] The patient was brought into the procedure room and placed in the prone position on the fluoroscopy table. An intravenous infusion of **[Abx]** was started and completed over one hour. Standard monitors were placed and vital signs were observed throughout the procedure. The area of the **[cervical/thoracic/lumbar]** spine was prepped with alcohol times three, then Hibiclens times three, then betadine scrub times three then betadine paint times three and draped in a sterile manner. The surgical site was covered with an Ioban covering.

The **[XX-XX]** interspace was identified. The skin and subcutaneous tissues in the area were anesthetized with 1% lidocaine. A 14-gauge Tuohy epidural needle was advanced with a paramedian approach from the **[right/left]** using a loss of resistance technique with a glass syringe and air in order to identify entrance into the epidural space. Once a good loss of resistance was obtained, negative aspiration was confirmed. An **[8]** contact lead was advanced under fluoroscopic guidance until the 0-position was at **[upper/mid/lower XX vertebral body level]. [A second lead was placed using the same technique from the XX-XX interspace on the right/left until the 0-position was at the upper/mid/lower XX vertebral body level.]** The leads were connected to an external trial programmer using sterile connectors. Several combinations of lead configuration, frequency, amplitude, and pulse width were used until comfortable and appropriate coverage of the patient's pain area was obtained.

SCS Implantation (*Continued*)

An incision was marked along the spine, which would allow exposure of the needle(s). The skin and subcutaneous tissues were anesthetized with 1% lidocaine. The skin incision was made with a scalpel, then extended to the supraspinous ligament using electrocautery. Hemostasis was well obtained with electrocautery. The needle(s) were then carefully removed and the lead(s) were secured to the supraspinous ligament with **[modified chest tube ties]** and 2-0 silk suture. Fluoroscopy was used to confirm continued proper placement of the lead(s) after being anchored.

A site was chosen for placement of the IPG unit in the **[right/left]** upper buttock area, below the belt line. An incision was marked and then the skin and subcutaneous tissues in the area were anesthetized with 1% lidocaine. A scalpel was used for the skin incision. The incision was extended with electrocautery to about 2 cm deep into the subcutaneous tissue. Blunt dissection was used to create an appropriately sized pocket. Hemostasis was well obtained with electrocautery.

A track for the extension to connect the lead(s) to the IPG unit was marked, then anesthetized with 1% lidocaine. A tunneling rod was used to create the track, going from the lead insertion site to the IPG unit site. The lead(s) were then placed through the rod and pulled into the pocket site. Extensions were then connected to the lead(s) and tightened with a hex wrench. The extensions were covered with a plastic bootie and secured with silk ties. The lead extensions were then connected to the IPG device with a hex wrench. Fluoroscopy confirmed continued proper placement of the lead(s) after the final connections were made.

Both incision sites were irrigated with antibiotic solution. Excess lead was placed deep to the IPG unit in the pocket site. The subcutaneous tissues were closed with 2-0 vicryl in an interrupted manner. The skin closure was done with **[staples OR subcuticular stitches using 2-0 vicryl]**. After the subcuticular closure was complete, steri-strips were used to maintain the closure. The ChloraPrep was then cleaned off the skin. Dressings consisted of **[xeroform, gauze, Tegaderm OR other]**.

The serial numbers for the leads and IPG unit are: **[XXXXXXXXXXX]**. The manufacturer and representative present were: **[XXXXXXXXXX]**.

Disposition: The patient tolerated the procedure well and there were no apparent complications. Vital signs remained stable throughout the procedure. The patient was taken to the recovery area where written discharge instructions for the procedure were given. **[POSTOP PLAN IS ...]** **[return to clinic in 7 days for staple removal/Postoperative check ...]**.

Infusion Pump Refill/Reprogramming

Patient Name: MR#: Date of Procedure:
Preoperative Diagnosis: **[XXXXXX]**
Postoperative Diagnosis: **[XXXXXX]**

Operation Title:
1) Electronic Analysis and reprogramming of infusion pump;
2) Refill and maintenance of infusion pump

Attending Physician:
Assistant Physician:
Anesthesia: **[local]**

Indications: The patient is a **[age]** old **[male/female]** with a diagnosis of **[XXXXX]**. The patient's history and physical exam have been reviewed. The risks, benefits, and alternatives to the procedure have been discussed, and all questions have been answered to the patient's satisfaction. The patient agreed to proceed and written informed consent was obtained.

Procedure in Detail: The patient was brought into the procedure room and placed on the gurney for the procedure. Interrogation was performed and revealed the following settings:

Drug/Concentration: **[drug @ XX mg/mL or mcg/mL]**

Infusion Mode/Rate: **[simple continuous @ XX mg/day or mcg/day];** Reservoir Volume: **[XX]**; Low Reservoir Alarm Date: **[date]**

The pump site was then prepped with chloroprep times three and draped with sterile towels. The refill template was placed over the pump and the refill port was located. A 22-gauge Huber needle with clamped tubing attached was advanced into the refill port. A **[XX mL]** syringe was attached, the tubing unclamped, and aspiration was steady until bubbles were noted.

[[XX] mL were withdrawn versus [xx] mL were expected.] The tubing was then reclamped and a new syringe containing **[XX mL]** of **[drug @ XX mg/mL or mcg/mL]** was attached. The tubing was then unclamped and the pump was filled easily without overpressure. After reclamping the tube, the needle was then removed, the area cleaned, and a bandage placed over the site of needle insertion. After reprogramming, the following settings were noted:

Drug/Concentration: **[drug @ XX mg/mL or mcg/mL];** Infusion Mode/ Rate: **[simple continuous @ XX mg/day or mcg/day];** Reservoir Volume: **[XX]**; Low Reservoir Alarm Date: **[date]**

Disposition: The patient tolerated the procedure well, and there were no apparent complications. Vital signs remained stable throughout the procedure. The patient was taken to the recovery area where written discharge instructions for the procedure were given. **[POSTOP PLAN IS ...]**

Intrathecal Trial

Patient Name: MR#: Date of Procedure:
Preoperative Diagnosis: **[diagnosis]**
Postoperative Diagnosis: **[diagnosis]**

Operation Title:
1) Intrathecal Catheter Placement; 2) Intraoperative Fluoroscopy;
3) **[IV Conscious Sedation]**

Attending Physician:
Assistant Physician:
Anesthesia: Local **[and conscious sedation with ...]**

Indications: The patient is a **[age]** old **[male/female]** with a diagnosis of **[diagnosis]**. The patient's history and physical exam were reviewed. The risks, benefits, and alternatives to the procedure have been discussed; all questions were answered to the patient's satisfaction. The patient agreed to proceed and written informed consent was obtained.

Procedure in Detail: [An IV was started while the patient was in the preoperative holding area.] The patient was brought into the procedure room and placed in the prone position on the fluoroscopy table. Standard monitors were placed and vital signs were observed throughout the procedure. The area of the **[lumbar]** spine was prepped with chloroprep times three and draped in a sterile manner.

The **[XX-XX]** interspace was identified and marked under AP fluoroscopy. The skin and subcutaneous tissues in the area were anesthetized with 1% lidocaine. A 20-gauge Tuohy epidural needle was directed toward the interspace under fluoroscopic guidance until the dura mater was punctured. This location was confirmed by the free flow of CSF. A 24-gauge catheter was advanced into the intrathecal space under fluoroscopic guidance to the **[XX]** vertebral level.

The patient's back was cleaned and the catheter was secured to the patient's back with a Tegaderm dressing and tape. Once the catheter was secured, **[XX mg/mcg]** of **[opioid/baclofen]** was administered and then flushed with 1 mL of preservative-free normal saline.

Disposition: The patient tolerated the procedure well and there were no apparent complications. Vital signs remained stable throughout the procedure. The patient was taken to the recovery area where **[he/she]** will be admitted for a 23-hour observation

Intrathecal Catheter and Infusion Pump Implantation

Patient Name: MR#: Date of Procedure:
Preoperative Diagnosis: **[diagnosis]**
Postoperative Diagnosis: **[diagnosis]**

Operation Title:
1) Intrathecal Catheter Implantation; 2) Programmable infusion pump implantation for subarachnoid drug delivery; 3) Intraoperative Fluoroscopy

Attending Physician:
Assistant Physician:
Anesthesia: General ET Anesthesia

Indications: The patient is a **[age]** old **[male/female]** with a diagnosis of **[diagnosis]**. The patient is here today for implantation of an intrathecal catheter and programmable infusion pump. The patient's history and physical exam were reviewed. The risks, benefits, and alternatives to the procedure have been discussed; all questions were answered to the patient's satisfaction. The patient agreed to proceed and written informed consent was obtained.

Procedure in Detail: [An IV was started while the patient was in the preoperative holding area.] The patient was brought into the procedure room and placed in the supine position on the fluoroscopy table. Standard monitors were placed and vital signs were observed throughout the procedure. An antibiotic infusion of **[abx]** was started and completed in over one hour. After induction of general anesthesia, the patient was turned to the **[right/left]** lateral decubitus position. The area of the **[thoracolumbar]** spine was prepped with alcohol times three, then Hibiclens times three, then ChloraPrep scrub times three, then ChloraPrep paint times three, and draped in a sterile manner.

The **[XX-XX]** interspace was identified and marked under AP fluoroscopy. The skin and subcutaneous tissues in the area were anesthetized with 1% lidocaine. A 15-gauge Tuohy epidural needle was directed toward the interspace under fluoroscopic guidance until the dura mater was punctured. This location was confirmed by the free flow of CSF. A 5 cm vertical incision was marked above the noted interspace and was made after additional skin infiltration with 1% lidocaine. The incision was extended with electrocautery to the supraspinous ligament. Hemostasis was well obtained. A purse string suture of 2-0 silk was placed around the needle. The needle was then carefully removed over the catheter, and the purse string was tied down. Continued flow of CSF was confirmed.

Intrathecal Catheter and Infusion Pump Implantation
(*Continued*)

A subcutaneous pocket was created for placement of the infusion pump in the **[right/left]** lower quadrant of the abdomen. The skin and subcutaneous tissues in the area were anesthetized with 1% lidocaine. A scalpel was used for the skin incision. The incision was extended with electrocautery to about 2 cm deep in the subcutaneous tissue. Blunt dissection was used to create an appropriately sized pocket for the infusion pump. Hemostasis was well obtained with electrocautery.

A track for the tunnel to connect the catheter to the infusion pump was marked and then anesthetized with 1% lidocaine. A tunneling rod was used to create the track, going from the pump pocket site to the catheter site. The catheter was then placed through the rod and pulled into the pocket site. Continued flow of CSF was confirmed.

The pump was primed and filled with **[XX mg/mcg of DRUG with a concentration of XX mg/mL]**. The catheter was trimmed by 1 inch and then attached and secured to the connector with 2-0 silk. The "nipple" connector was then snapped onto the pump and secured with 2-0 silk. The pocket was irrigated thoroughly with antibiotic solution; hemostasis was again confirmed. Excess catheter was carefully coiled and placed deep to the pump in the pocket site.

The spine incision was also irrigated with antibiotic solution. Both incisions were closed at the subcutaneous layer with 2-0 vicryl interrupted suture. The skin closure was done with **[staples OR subcuticular stitches using 2-0 vicryl]**. After the subcuticular closure was complete, steri-strips were used to maintain the closure. The ChloraPrep was then cleaned off the skin. Dressings consisted of **[xeroform, gauze, Tegaderm OR other]**. The patient was then allowed to emerge from general anesthesia.

The serial number for the infusion pump unit is: **[XXXXXXXXXXXX]**. The manufacturer and representative present were: **[XXXXXXXXXXX]**.

Disposition: The patient was returned to a supine position and transferred to the recovery room on a gurney. The patient tolerated the procedure well and there were no apparent complications. Vital signs remained stable throughout the procedure. Written discharge instructions for the procedure were given. **[POSTOP PLAN IS ...] [Return to clinic in 7 days for staple removal/Postoperative check ...]**

Current Pump Settings: [DRUG/CONCENTRATION; RESERVOIR VOLUME; INFUSION MODE; DAILY/HOURLY RATE; ALARM DATE].

Suggested SCS Lead Placement

Level	Coverage
C2, C3	Occipital Neuralgia, Cervical Postlaminectomy, Axial Neck Pain
C4	Shoulder blades, Rhomboid, Shoulder Joint
C5, C6	Upper extremity pain, Hands, Arms, Peripheral Neuropathy
C7	Hands, CRPS
T2, T3	Intractable Angina
T4, T5	Post-thoracotomy, Post-mastectomy, Post-herpetic Neuralgia (chest wall)
T6, T7	Pancreatitis
T8, T9	Low Back Pain, Lumbar Postlaminectomy Syndrome, Axial Low Back Pain
T10, T11	Lumbar Radiculopathy, Restless Leg Syndrome
T12	Groin (off-midline), Foot (midline)
S2	Genitals, Rectum, Pelvis, Inguinal Neuralgia, Hernia
S3	Vulvadynia, Endometriosis

Intrathecal Pump: Catheter Dye Study

1. Use Medtronic Model 8540 Catheter Access Port (CAP) Kit to access the catheter access port septum.

2. Aspirate approximately 1 mL of fluid from the catheter access port to ensure removal of drug from the catheter access port and catheter. **If complete kink/occlusion has occurred, aspiration from the catheter access port may be impossible. If partial occlusion has occurred, aspiration may be difficult.

3. Inject at least 1 mL of imaging solution into the catheter access port using a 10 mL (or larger) syringe. If partial occlusion or occlusion has occurred, do NOT force injection (can bolus patient by accident).

4. Evaluate the catheter and delivery site as follows: Since the contrast medium will diffuse rapidly throughout the CSF for intrathecal catheters, elevating the head of the x-ray table will enhance caudal diffusion of the solution. For epidural catheters, the contrast medium will diffuse more slowly and remain localized. **If complete kink/occlusion has occurred, injection of contrast medium through the access port will be impossible. If a partial occlusion has occurred, injection will be difficult.

5. Flush contrast medium through the catheter and catheter access system with at least 1 mL of sterile preservative-free sodium chloride for injection.

6. If the catheter is patent, intact, and in place, program a bolus equal to the calculated volume of fluid in the catheter, from the pump connector to the catheter tip.

7. To diffuse drug, program the desired prescription.

8. If the catheter is kinked, disconnected, or dislodged, it should be surgically repaired.

9. If the catheter has migrated, surgical revision or dose adjustment may be necessary.

New Patient Billing and Coding

LEVEL 1: NON-PHYSICIAN VISIT
NEW PATIENTS: ALL THREE* AREAS MUST BE MET FOR
CODING AND BILLING

	Level 5	Level 4	Level 3	Level 2
Code: New OR Consult	99205 new 99245 consult	99204 99244	99203 99243	99202 99242
Chief complaint	Required	Required	Required	Required
*HPI	4	4	4	1
ROS	10	10	2	1
PFSH	3	3	1	0
*PE	2 elements from 9 areas/ systems	2 elements from 9 areas/ systems	>2 elements from 6 areas or >12 elements from 2 areas	>6 elements
*Decision making†	High complexity	Moderate complexity	Limited	Straight-forward

Elements of HPI
Location:
Severity:
Quality:
Duration:
Timing:
Context:
Associated Signs and Symptoms:
Modifying Factors:

PE Areas/Systems
Please refer to Dictation Templates

---

*CONSULTATIONS must state referring MD and MD must be sent a copy of the dictated report (include address).

†Greater than **[XX]** minutes spent discussing... with this patient....

Follow-Up Patient Billing and Coding

LEVEL 1: NON-PHYSICIAN VISIT
NEW PATIENTS: TWO OF THE THREE* AREAS MUST BE MET FOR CODING AND BILLING.

	Level 5	Level 4	Level 3	Level 2
Code:	99215	99214	99213	99212
Chief complaint	Required	Required	Required	Required
*HPI	4	4	1	1
ROS	10	2	1	0
PFSH	2	1	N/A	0
*PE	2 elements from 9 areas/ systems	2 elements from 6 areas/systems OR >12 elements from 2 areas	>6 elements	1–5 elements
*Decision making†	High complexity	Moderate complexity	Low complexity	Straight-forward

Elements of HPI
Location:
Severity:
Quality:
Duration:
Timing:
Context:
Associated Signs and Symptoms:
Modifying Factors:

PE Areas/Systems
Please refer to Dictation Templates.

---

*CONSULTATIONS must state referring MD and MD must be sent a copy of the dictated report (include address).

†Greater than **[XX]** minutes were spent discussing... with this patient....

Regional Landmarks

Block	Elbow	Wrist
Radial	Between biceps tendon and brachioradialis muscle in AC fossa	Lateral (radial) to the radial artery
Ulnar	Between olecranon and medial epicondyle above level of elbow to avoid direct nerve trauma	Medial (ulnar) to ulnar artery
Median	Medial to brachial artery between the 2 heads of the pronator teres	Between FCR and palmaris longus

Femoral: Lateral to femoral artery (NAVL)

Sciatic: Patient in lateral decubitus position with HF & KF: Connect PSIS & GT: At midpoint, drop perpendicular 3 cm as target.

Lateral Femoral Cutaneous: Vulnerable to compression at iliac spine where it passes btwn bone and attachment of the sartorius muscle. ASIS: 2 cm medial/2 cm inferior, below inguinal ligament.

Ilioinguinal: ASIS: 3 cm medial/3 cm inferior, above inguinal ligament.

Genitofemoral: Just lateral to pubic tubercle.

*Tarsal tunnel is posterior and inferior to the medial malleolus (MM).

Lateral Border = Tibia; Medial Border = Flexor Retinaculum (lancinate)

*Tarsal Tunnel Members: Tibial N, Posterior Tibialis, EDL, FHL, Tibial A/V

Tibial: Posterior to MM

Saphenous: Anterior to MM

Sural: Posterior to LM

Superficial peroneal: Anterior to LM: Draw a line connecting the MM & lateral malleolus (LM) and place a cuff of anesthesia around it.

Vertebral Levels

Fibers	Termination
Conus medullaris (caudal tip of SC)	L1-L2
Subarachnoid; subdural space	S1-S3
Filum terminale	Sacral hiatus (S5-Coccyx)
Epidural venous plexus	S4

Brachial Plexus

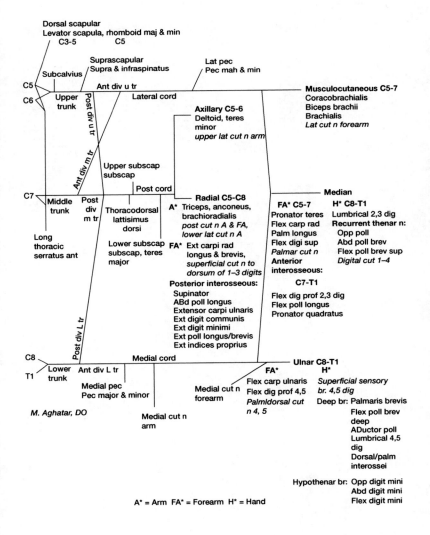

Dorsal scapular
Levator scapula, rhomboid maj & min
C3-5   C5

Suprascapular   Lat pec
Supra & infraspinatus Pec mah & min

Subclavius

C5   Ant div u tr   Musculocutaneous C5-7
C6   Upper   Lateral cord   Coracobrachialis
     trunk   Biceps brachii
                                         Brachialis
                                         Lat cut n forearm

Post div u tr

Axillary C5-6
Deltoid, teres
minor
upper lat cut n arm

Ant div m tr

Upper subscap
subscap

Post cord

C7   Middle   Post   Radial C5-C8   Median
     trunk   div   A* Triceps, anconeus,   FA* C5-7   H* C8-T1
              m tr   Thoracodorsal   brachioradialis   Pronator teres Lumbrical 2,3 dig
                     lattisimus   *post cut n A & FA,* Flex carp rad   Recurrent thenar n:
Long   dorsi   *lower lat cut n A*   Palm longus   Opp poll
thoracic   Flex digi sup   Abd poll brev
serratus ant   Lower subscap FA* Ext carpi rad   *Palmar cut n*   Flex poll brev sup
                     subscap, teres   longus & brevis,   Anterior   *Digital cut 1-4*
                     major   *superficial cut n to* interosseous:
                                        dorsum of 1-3 digits   C7-T1

                                        Posterior interosseous: Flex dig prof 2,3 dig
                                        Supinator   Flex poll longus
                                        ABd poll longus   Pronator quadratus
                                        Extensor carpi ulnaris
                                        Ext digit communis
                                        Ext digit minimi
                                        Ext poll longus/brevis
                                        Ext indices proprius

Post div L tr

C8   Medial cord   Ulnar C8-T1
T1   Lower   Ant div L tr   FA*   H*
     trunk   Flex carp ulnaris   *Superficial sensory*
     Medial pec   Medial cut n   Flex dig prof 4,5   *br. 4,5 dig*
     Pec major & minor   forearm   *Palm/dorsal cut*   Deep br: Palmaris brevis
                                             n 4, 5   Flex poll brev
M. Aghatar, DO   deep
                         Medial cut n   ADuctor poll
                         arm   Lumbrical 4,5
                                                                          dig
                                                                          Dorsal/palm
                                                                          interossei

                                             Hypothenar br: Opp digit mini
                                                            Abd digit mini
                         A* = Arm FA* = Forearm H* = Hand   Flex digit mini

Brachial Plexopathies

Characteristics	Radiation	Tumor
Site of Injury	Upper trunk	Lower trunk
Clinical Presentations	Myokymia	Horner's Syndrome
Sensation	Painless	Painful

Lumbosacral Plexus

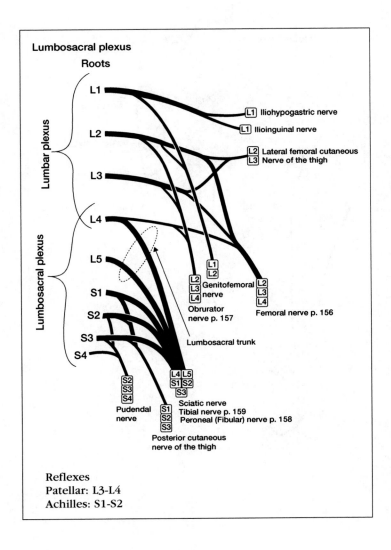

Lumbosacral plexus

Roots

L1
L2
L3
L4
L5
S1
S2
S3
S4

Lumbar plexus

Lumbosacral plexus

L1 Iliohypogastric nerve
L1 Ilioinguinal nerve
L2 Lateral femoral cutaneous
L3 Nerve of the thigh

L1
L2 Genitofemoral nerve
L2
L3
L4

Obrurator nerve p. 157

L2
L3
L4 Femoral nerve p. 156

Lumbosacral trunk

S2
S3
S4
Pudendal nerve

L4 L5
S1 S2
S3
Sciatic nerve
Tibial nerve p. 159
Peroneal (Fibular) nerve p. 158

S1
S2
S3
Posterior cutaneous nerve of the thigh

Reflexes
Patellar: L3-L4
Achilles: S1-S2

Femoral Nerve

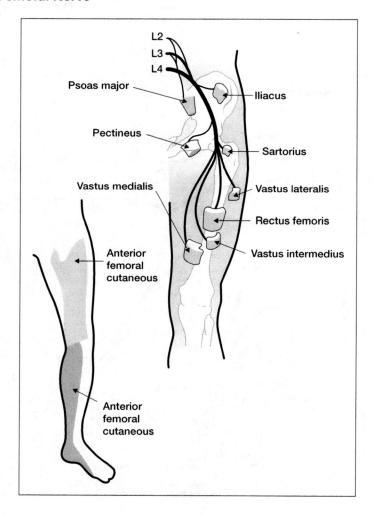

Obturator Nerve

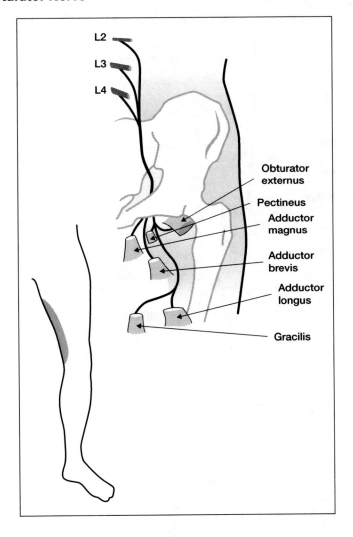

Peroneal (Fibular) Nerve

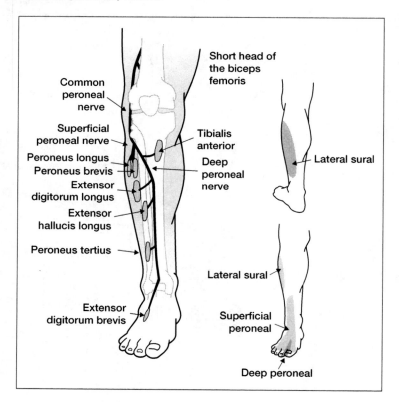

Tibial Nerve

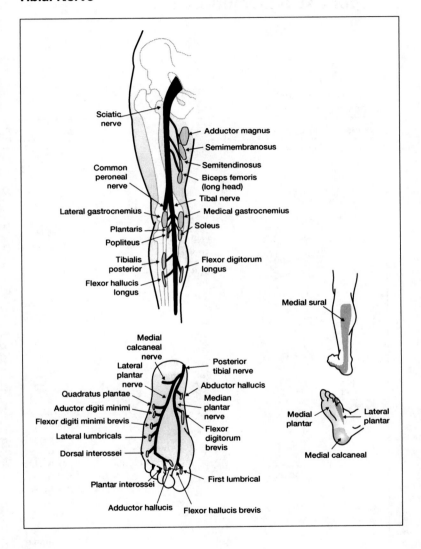

Upper Extremity Innervations

Biceps reflex: C5-6
Brachioradialis reflex: C5-6
Triceps reflex: C7-8

Roots	M-C	Axillary	Radial	Median	Ulnar
C5-6	Biceps brachialis	Deltoid T. minor	Supinator		
C5-6-C7	Coraco-brachialis		Brachio-radialis		
C6-7				Pronator Teres FCR	
C7-6-C7-8			ECR Longus Triceps		
C7-8			ECR Brevis Ext. Dig. EIP, EDM, ECU Abd. Poll. Longus Ext. Poll. Brevis Ext. Poll. Longus	Palmaris Longus	FCU
C7-8-T1			Anconeus	FDS (4)	
C8-T1				FDP (2) FPL, Pronator Quad., Lumbricals (2), Opponens Poll, Abd. P. Brevis, Flex P. Brevis (1/2)	FDP (2) Dorsal Interossei (4) Palmar Interossei (3) Lumbricals (2) Add. Poll, Flex P. Brevis (1/2), Hypothenar muscles, Palmaris Brevis

Lower Extremity Innervations

Femoral N	Obturator N	Superior Gluteal N	Inferior Gluteal N
Sartorius	Ob. Externus	TFL (L4-5)	Glut. Max
(L2-3) Iliacus	(L3-4) Pectineus	Glut. Med (L5-S1)	(L5-S1-S2)
(L2-3)	(L2-3)	Glut. Min	
Pectineus	Add. Brevis	(L5-S1-S2)	
(L2-3)	(L2-3-4)		
Quads: (L2-3–4):	Add. Longus		
V. Medialis	(L2-3-4) Gracilis		
V. Intermed.	(L2-3)		
V. Lateralis			
Rectus			
Femoris			

Sciatic N: Peroneal Division	Sciatic N: Tibial Division	Common Peroneal N Deep PN	Tibial N
Biceps Femoris:	Semimembranosus	EDL (L5-S1)	Gastrocnemius (S1-2)
Short Head (L5-S1-S2)	(L5-S1-S2)	Tib. Ant. (L4-5) EHL (L5-S1)	Plantaris (S1-2) Soleus
	Semitendonosus (L5-S1-S2)	Per. Tertius (L5-S1)	(S1-2) Popliteus (L4-5-S1)
	Biceps Femoris: Long Head	EDB (L5-S1)	Post Tib N
	(L5-S1-S2) Add. Magnus (L4)	SF PN	Tib. Post (L4-5) FDL (S2-3)
		Peroneus Longus (L5-S1)	FHL (S2-3)
		Peroneus Brevis (L5-S1)	Med Plantar N
			FDB (S2-3) Abd Hall Brevis (S2-3) FHB (S2-3) 1st Lumbrical (S2-3)
			Lat Plantar N (all S2-3)
			Abd Dig Min Quad Plantae FDM-Brevis 2-4 Lumbricals Interossei Abd Hall

PM&R/Neurology Exam Guide

Reflex Score	Definition
1+	Hyporeflexic
2+	Normoreflexic
3+	Hyperreflexic
4+	Crossover/clonus

UMN	Spasticity hypertonic hyperreflexic dermatomal sensory
LMN	Hypo/normotonic hyporeflexic peripheral or dermatomal sensory

MANUAL MOTOR TESTING

1+	2+	3+	4+	5+
Trace movement: flicker of contraction	Movement with gravity (in same plane)	Movement against gravity without resistance: with full ROM	Movement against gravity with partial resistance	Movement against gravity with full resistance

Score	Modified Ashworth Score Definition
0	No increase in muscle tone
1	Slight increase in tone with catch or release or minimal resistance at end of range
2	Slight increase in tone with catch or release and with minimal resistance through range following catch
3	More marked increased tone throughout ROM
4	Considerable increase in tone; passive movement difficult
5	Affected part rigid

Dermatomes

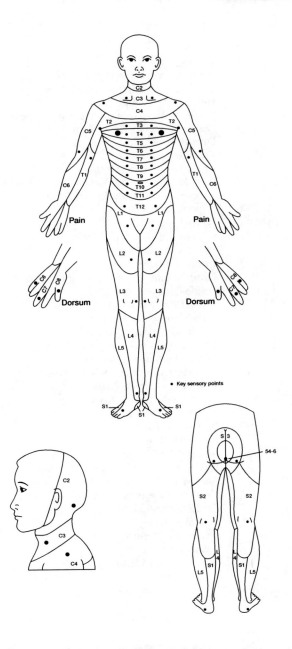

Key sensory points

Physical Exam Tests and Acronyms

AKA	Above Knee Amputation
A/P ROM	Active/Passive Range Of Motion
BKA	Below Knee Amputation
cADLs	Community Activities of Daily Living
DIP	Distal Interphalangeal Joint
DRG	Dorsal Root Ganglion
EMG	Electromyography
ESI	Epidural Steroid Injection
FABER	Flexion, Abduction, External Rotation (Patrick)
FAIR	Flexion, Adduction, Internal Rotation
GENU VALGUS	"Knock-Kneed"
GENU VARUS	"Bow-Legged"
GTB	Greater Trochanteric Bursa/Bursitis
IAP	Inferior Articular Process
IPG	Implantable Pulse Generator
KEMP'S	Lumbar Extension & Torsional Stress (Traditionally Loads Facet Joints)
MBB	Medial Branch Block
NCS	Nerve Conduction Study
pADLs	Personal Activities of Daily Living
PIP	Proximal Interphalangeal Joint
RFA	Radiofrequency Ablation
R-SLR	Reverse Straight Leg Raise (Stresses L1, L2 (L3) Roots)
RW	Rolling Walker (Rollator)
SAP	Superior Articular Process
SC	Straight Cane
SCI	Spinal Cord Injury
SIJ	Sacroiliac Joint
SLR	Straight Leg Raise (Stresses (L3), L4, L5 and S1-2 Roots)
SLUMP	Seated Version of SLR (Hip Flexion; KE)
SPURLING	Cervical Extension & Torsional Stress (Traditionally Loads Facet Joints; Compresses Neural Foramen)
TBI	Traumatic Brain Injury
TP	Transverse Process
TPI	Trigger Point Injection
WC	Wheelchair

Therapy Contraindications

Chiropractic Spinal Manipulation Contraindications:
Malignancy involving the spinal column/meninges/spine. Aggressive benign tumor, acute fracture, dislocation of vertebra, spondylolisthesis, acute infection of the spine, RA, AS, recent Fx, spinal surgery within last 6 months, radiculopathy with progressive neurological signs, Arnold–Chiari malformation, internal fixation/stabilization devices, sign of instability, positive Kernig–Lhermitte sign, cauda equina lesion, congenital, generalized hypermobility, syringomyelia, diastematomyelia, aneurysm near site of manipulation, vertebrobasilar insufficiency, osteopenia or osteoporosis

Source: WHO Guidelines on Basic Training and Safety in Chiropractic, 2005.

Acupuncture Contraindications:
Severe bleeding diathesis, systemic sepsis, cellulitis, burns, ulceration. First Trimester, anticoagulation
Acupuncture Mediated By:
1–2 Hz: Enkephalins and enorphin release
@ 100 Hz: Dynorphin

Source: Wilkinson J, Faleiro R. Acupuncture in Pain Management. Continuing Education in Anesthesia, Critical Care & Pain.

TENS Contraindications:
Implanted pacemaker, history of heart disease, discontinue if irritation of skin. Do not use in transthoracic area. Be cautious in areas of impaired sensation, skin lesions, atrophic skin, and dermatitis.

Avoid stimulation over the carotid sinuses and anterior aspect of neck.

Avoid allergy to gel or electrodes. Controversy in use during pregnancy.

Source: 1. Knight KL, Draper DO. Application Procedures: Electrotherapy. Therapeutic Modalities: The Art and Science. 2. www.electrotherapy.org/modalities/transcutaneous-electrical-nerve-stimulation-tens

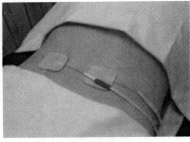

TENS SET UP

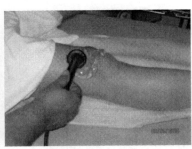

ULTRASOUND TO THE KNEE

P&O Reference

Orthosis Clinical Indication

Spinomed Orthosis	Thoracic/lumbar compression fx
Thoracolumbar Corset	Thoracic/lumbar chronic LBP
Hyperextension Orthosis	Thoracic/lumbar compression fx
Chairback Orthosis	Lumbar stenosis; HNP; strain/sprain
LSO–Pull Cord Design	Lumbar stenosis; HNP; strain/sprain
Lumbosacral Corset	LBP, lumbar stenosis; strain/sprain
Elastic Lumbosacral Binder	LBP, lumbar stenosis; strain/sprain
Sacroiliac Orthosis	Sacroiliac Dysfunction
Plantar Fasciitis Night Splint	Plantar Fasciitis, Achilles tendinitis
Air Stirrup Ankle Orthosis	Medial/Lateral ankle instability, ankle sprain/strain
Cock Up Wrist Splint (Neutral)	CTS, wrist sprain/strain
Thumb Spica Splint	CTS, OA (especially 1st CMC)
Tennis Elbow Strap	Medial/Lateral Epicondylosis
Heelbo Elbow Pad	Ulnar Neuropathy
Genumedi Elbow Sleeve	Medial/Lateral Epicondylosis, Ulnar Neuropathy

Research Critical Appraisal Questions

1. What is the research question?
   (Is the paper concerned with the impact of an intervention, causality, or determining the magnitude of a health problem?)

2. *Is this an important research question? Are important related questions left unaddressed?*

3. What is the study type?
   (retrospective vs prospective; observational vs intervention; etc.)

4. Is the study type appropriate to the research question? If not, how useful are the results produced by the study design?

5. What are the outcome factors (end points, dependent variables) and how are they measured?

6. Are all relevant outcomes assessed? Is there measurement error?
   In an experimental study: Are the assessors of outcomes blind to group assignment?

7. How important are omitted outcomes? Is measure error or bias an important source of bias?

8. What are the study factors (interventions, independent variables, predictors) and how are they measured?

9. Are all relevant study factors assessed? Is there measurement error?

10. Is measure error an important source of bias?

11. What important potential confounders are considered?

12. Are potential confounders controlled for? Are there confounders that were not controlled for?

13. Is confounding (whatever is left after statistical and other controls) an important source of bias?

14. What are the sampling frame (population) and sampling method? What is the sample size? Are potential confounders controlled for?

15. Is there selection bias?

16. Does this threaten the external validity of the study?

17. *In an experimental study*: How were the subjects assigned to groups?
    In a longitudinal study: How many reached the final follow-up?
    In a case-control study: Are the controls appropriate?
    In an experimental study: Is there assignment bias?

18. *In all studies*: Was attrition selective?

19. Does this threaten the internal validity of the study?

20. Are statistical tests used?

21. Are the tests appropriate to the data? Are confidence intervals given? Are effect sizes given? If a null result: Is the power given? Was the sample size adequate to detect a clinically/socially important result?

22. What are the results?

23. Are the results relevant to the research question(s)? Are there research questions for which no results are provided?

24. Are the results clinically/socially significant?

25. Is the effect or difference found clinically/socially relevant? Is the study useful or is the result inconclusive?

26. What conclusions did the authors reach about the study question? Are the conclusions based on the findings?

27. What claims for the applicability of the findings outside the sample studied do the authors make?

28. Is generalization justified on statistical bases? Logical bases? What exceptions might exist? Do the results apply to the population in which you are interested?

Sample Procedure Log Form

Procedure	ACGME Requirement	1st Quarter	2nd Quarter	3rd Quarter	4th Quarter	Total
Image-Guided Spinal Injection: Cervical	15					
Image-Guided Spinal Injection: Lumbar	20					
Injection of Major Joint or Bursa	10					
Trigger Point Injections	20					
Sympathetic Blockade	10					
Neurolytic Technique, Including Chemical and RFA	5					
Spinal Cord Stimulation	3					
Placement of Permanent Spinal Drug Delivery System	3					

Sample Patient Safety Log

Date/Time	Event & Outcome	Plan for Improvement System-Based Practice Model

Pain Scale Reference

		2	3	4	5	6	7	8	9	10
Verbal Description Pain	No Pain	Mild Pain		Moderate Pain			Severe Pain			Worst Pain Possible
Wong-Baker Facial Grimace Scale*	Face 0 is very happy because he or she doesn't hurt at all.	Face 2 hurts just a little bit.		Face 4 hurts a little more.		Face 6 hurts even more.		Face 8 hurts a whole lot.		Face 10 hurts as much as you can imagine, although you don't have to be crying to feel this bad.
Activity Tolerance Scale	No Pain	Can be ignored		Interferes with tasks and concentration			Interferes with basic needs			Bedrest Required

*The Wong-Baker Facial Grimace Scale is commonly used for pediatric patients and can be found at wongbakerfaces.org

Resources

Regional Websites
www.nysora.com
www.asra.com

Organizations
International Spine Interventional Society: ISIS
APS: American Pain Society
AAPMR: American Academy of PM&R: www.aapmr.org
ABA: American Board of Anesthesiology: www.theaba.org
American Society of Regional Anesthesia and Pain Medicine: ASRA
American Academy of Pain Medicine: AAPM
American Board of Pain Medicine: ABPM
International Association for the Study of Pain: IASP

ACGME Training Standards

ACGME FELLOWSHIP REQUIREMENTS

Neurology	▨ 15 complete neurological examinations, including MSE, CN, MME, Sensory Exam, Reflex, Cerebellar, Gait examinations (5 supervised by faculty) ▨ OR Residency Completion
Neuroradiology	▨ 15 MRI/CT evaluations: brain, cervical, thoracic, and/or lumbar spine
PM&R	▨ 15 complete musculoskeletal and neuromuscular history and examinations including: static/dynamic flexibility, strength, coordination, agility ▨ Clinical evaluation and rehabilitation plan development in 5 cases ▨ OR Residency Completion
Psychiatry	▨ 15 complete MSE with assessment for personality d/o (5 supervised by faculty) ▨ OR Residency Completion
Anesthesiology	▨ 15 IV access + basic airway management, mask ventilation, endotracheal intubations + direct management of sedation ▨ Proficiency in ACLS and BLS ▨ 15 administration of neuraxial analgesia with interlaminar technique ▨ OR Residency Completion
Outpatient Chronic Non-Cancer Pain	▨ 50 different patients followed for at least 2 months ▨ 25 patients undergoing interventional pain procedures
Inpatient Chronic Pain	▨ 15 new-patient consults
Inpatient Acute Pain	▨ 50 new-patient consults
Cancer Pain	▨ 20 different patients
Palliative Care	▨ 10 patients, longitudinal involvement
Pediatric Pain	▨ Suggested (5 patients)

ACGME FELLOWSHIP PROCEDURE REQUIREMENTS

Intervention	Procedures
Minimum Total Interventional Procedures	60
Image-Guided Spinal Intervention Techniques—Cervical Spine	15
Image-Guided Spinal Intervention Techniques—Lumbar Spine	25
Neuroablative Procedures	10
Injection of Major Joint or Bursa	5
Trigger Point Injections	10
Spinal Cord Stimulation	3
Intradiscal Procedures	10
Permanent Spinal Drug Delivery System	3
Sympathetic Blockade	10

▓ ACGME CORE COMPETENCIES

Medical Knowledge
READ
Recognize Patterns
Explain Patterns
Acquire New Knowledge
Demonstrate New Knowledge

Patient Care
PRIME
Prioritize Tasks
Report Data
Interpret Data
Manage Data
Educate: Yourself & Others

Practice-Based Learning and Improvement
FIRST
Find Evidence, Feedback
Information Use (Data Analysis)
Review & Reflect
Study & Share for Improvement
Teaching

Systems-Based Practice
TACTICS
Teamwork Advocacy Coordination
Technology Use in Practice Improvement Tools & Skills
Cost-Effectiveness
Safety

Professionalism
IHEAARD
Integrity
Honesty
Excellence Accountability Altruism
Respect
Duty

Interpersonal and Communication Skills
PLEASE
Perspective Taking
Listening
Encouraging Input
Accuracy
Sustaining Relationships
Explaining

ACGME CORE COMPETENCIES (Continued)

Patient Care
- Provide compassionate, appropriate, and effective patient care.
- Take a thorough history, perform musculoskeletal and neurological examinations.
- Provide a comprehensive evaluation, including those elements listed above; include laboratory and imaging study review and interpretation.
- Interact effectively with patients and their families.
- Demonstrate respect and care for individuals.
- Identify red flags.
- Formulate a differential diagnosis.
- Formulate a multimodal treatment plan based on the individual patient's history, expectations, and expected course of his/her condition.
- Work together with other members of our interdisciplinary healthcare team to optimize patient care and enhance quality of life.

Medical Knowledge
- Demonstrate knowledge about established and evolving biomedical, clinical, and cognate sciences and the application of this knowledge to patient care.
- Apply relevant scientific knowledge and reasoning to the practice of chronic pain management.
- Demonstrate sound knowledge of the anatomy, physiology, and pharmacology of pain medicine.
- Demonstrate how specific physical and psychological states affect the management of chronic pain patients.
- Understand recent developments in pain medicine.

Interpersonal and Communication Skills
- Demonstrate interpersonal and communication skills that result in effective information exchange and teaming with patients, their families, and professional associates.
- Discuss the utility, advantages, and potential disadvantages of different treatment options (pharmacologic, interventional, and behavioral).
- Create and sustain a therapeutic and ethically sound relationship with patients.
- Use effective listening skills to elicit appropriate clinical information.
- Work effectively with others in an interdisciplinary healthcare team.

■ ACGME CORE COMPETENCIES (*Continued*)

Professionalism
- Demonstrate a commitment to carrying out professional responsibilities.
- Demonstrate respect, compassion, and integrity.
- Respond to the needs of patients and those of society; understand that those supersede self-interest.
- Demonstrate accountability to patients, society, colleagues, our institution, and our profession.
- Demonstrate a commitment to excellence and ongoing professional development.
- Demonstrate a commitment to ethical principles pertaining to the provision or withholding of care, the confidentiality of patient information, informed consent, and business practices.
- Demonstrate your responsiveness to patient's culture, age, gender, and disabilities.

Practice-Based Learning
- Investigate and evaluate one's own patient care practices, appraise and assimilate scientific evidence, and improve patient care practices.
- Locate, appraise, and assimilate information and evidence from scientific studies related to their patients' healthcare problems.
- Assist in the teaching of residents and medical students.
- Apply the knowledge of study designs and statistical methods to the appraisal of clinical studies and other information on diagnostic and therapeutic effectiveness.
- Use information technology to manage information, access online medical information, and support one's own education.

Systems-Based Practice
- Demonstrate an awareness of and responsiveness to the larger context and system of healthcare and the ability to effectively call on system resources to provide care that is of optimal value.
- Understand how one's own patient care and other professional practices affect other healthcare professionals, the healthcare organization, and our larger society.
- Understand which activities affect system performance.
- Practice pain medicine within the context of this healthcare institution and in cooperation with other healthcare professionals.
- Practice cost-effective healthcare.
- Advocate for quality patient care and assist patients in dealing with system complexities.

▓ Know how to partner with healthcare managers and providers to assess, coordinate, and improve healthcare.

▓ Assume responsibility for interacting with healthcare services (social and home care services, physical therapy) and other providers (psychiatry, neurology, PM&R ...) for coordinating optimal patient care and authorization for coverage of appropriate pharmacologic and interventional therapeutics.

Sample Reading Assignments

A. Residents

Essentials of Pain Medicine, 3rd Edition; H. Benzon, 2011.

Wk	Junior Resident Rotation	Senior Resident Rotation
1 50 pgs	Chp 1: Anatomy & Physiology Chp 2: Neurochemistry Chp 3: Taxonomy Chp 4: Physical Exam Chp 5: Pain Assessment Chp 6: Psychological Testing Chp 7: *DSM-IV* Chp 8: Neurophysiologic Testing	Chp 38: Migraines & Cluster Chp 39: Tension Headaches Chp 40: Meningeal Puncture HA Chp 41: Cervicogenic HA Chp 42: Orofacial Pain Chp 43: Low Back Pain Chp 44: Epidural Injections Chp 45: Transforaminal ESI
2 50 pgs	Chp 9: Common Pathologies Chp 10: Disability Chp 11: Major Opioids Chp 12: Opioids Mild/Moderate Pain	Chp 46: Facet Syndromes Chp 47: Buttock Pain Chp 48: Myofascial Pain Chp 49: Fibromyalgia Chp 50: CRPS Terminology Chp 51: Postherpetic Neuralgia Chp 52: Phantom Pain
3 45 pgs	Chp 13: Risk Stratification Chp 14: Legal Issues Chp 15: Psychopharmacology Chp 16: Membrane Stabilizers Chp 17: NSAIDs	Chp 53: Central Pain Chp 54: Pelvic Pain Chp 55: Peripheral Neuropathy Chp 56: Nerve Entrapments Chp 57: Pain in Children Chp 58: Geriatric Pain
4 25 pgs	Chp 18: Myofascial Pain Chp 19: Interventional Pharmacology Chp 22: PM&R Approaches to Pain	Chp 23: Acupuncture Chp 24: Psychological Tx Chp 25: Substance Abuse

B. Fellows

Essentials of Pain Medicine, 3rd Edition; H. Benzon, 2011.

Month	Reading Assignment
July	Chapters 1–9
August	Chapters 10–18
September	Chapters 19–24
October	Chapters 25–33
November	Chapters 34–45
December	Chapters 46–56
January	Chapters 57–64
February	Chapters 65–72
March	Chapters 73–80
April	Board review
May	Board review
June	Board review

Other Suggested Reading Materials

**Musculoskeletal Physical Examination: An Evidence Based Approach*;
Gerard A Malanga & Scott F Nadler, 2006

**Image-Guided Spine Intervention*; D. Fenton, L. Czervionke, 2003

**Atlas of Image-Guided Intervention in Regional Anesthesia and Pain
Medicine*; J. Rathmell, 2006

Practice Guidelines: Spinal Diagnostic & Treatment Procedures;
International Spine Intervention Society, 2004

Pain Management; S. Waldman, 2007

**Essentials of Pain Management & Regional Anesthesia*; H. Benzon,
2004

Complications in Regional Anesthesia & Pain Management; J. Neal &
J. Rathmell, 2007

Essentials of Musculoskeletal Care; W. Greene, 2005

The Massachusetts General Hospital Handbook of Pain Management;
J. Ballantyne, 2006

**Psychiatry 2008 Edition; *Current Clinical Strategies*; R. Hahn, L. Albers,
C. Reist, 2008

Atlas of Uncommon Pain Syndromes; S. Waldman, 2008

Clinical Anatomy of the Lumbar Spine and Sacrum; N. Bogduk, 2005

Headache Medicine Questions and Answers; D. Jamieson, 2009

**Pain Review*; S. Waldman, 2009

Surface Anatomy for Clinical Needle Electromyography; H. Lee &
J. DeLisa, 2000

Manual of Nerve Conduction Studies; R. Buschbacher & N. Prahlow,
2006.

**Easy Injections*; L. Weiss et al., 2007

**Botulinum Toxin Injection Guide*; I. Odderson, 2008.

Goals and Objectives

RESIDENTS

1. Junior Resident Clinical Objectives

- Define axial and radicular pain.
- Explain common causes of mechanical low back pain—including muscle strain, discogenic disease, vertebral fracture (compression), myofascial pain syndrome, facet arthropathy (lumbar spondylosis), hip osteoarthritis, and sacroiliac dysfunction.
- Define nociceptive and neuropathic pain.
- List receptors involved in nociception and centralized pain.
- Define somatic and visceral pain.
- Discuss the principles and indications of diagnostic, psychological, and neurophysiologic testing. Understand when MRI is preferred over CT imaging; discuss when gadolinium is used.
- Discuss the principles and indications of physical medicine and rehabilitation (PM&R) approaches to pain management—including the use of occupational and physical therapy programs, orthotics use, and the use of the physical modalities.
- Understand the definition of and determination of disability.
- Describe some of the mechanisms of chronic pain.
- Understand pain and its relation to psychosocial issues.
- Understand pain and its relation to depression and other psychiatric illnesses.
- Explain the epidemiology of pain and its economic impact.
- Understand major opioid use in pain management.
- Understand minor opioid use in pain management.
- Understand adverse effects of opioid therapy—including addiction.
- Understand the use of adjunctive analgesic medications—including membrane stabilizers, antidepressants, NSAIDs, and antispasmodics.
- Explain which receptors are targeted with adjuvant use.
- Understand interventional pharmacology including local anesthetic toxicity and corticosteroid choice.

2. Junior Resident Skill Objectives

- Be able to conduct a basic evaluation of and manage a patient with chronic pain.
- Conduct a full pain history; include the location, radiation, duration, frequency, and pain onset. Include a pain description, alleviating and exacerbating factors, and associated symptoms.
- Conduct a full medical, social, and surgical history. Incorporate an appropriate review of systems into a full historical examination.
- Conduct a full musculoskeletal and neurological physical examination; include a cranial nerve exam, stance and gait inspection examination, cervical/lumbar range of motion, upper and lower extremity manual motor testing, sensory testing and reflex examination, and appropriate provocative and nerve tension testing.
- Explain manual motor testing grades.
- Explain reflex examination scores.
- Provide a thorough differential diagnosis of the chief complaint.
- Provide a hypothesis for the level of nerve root irritation (radiculopathy) based on the history (description of pain radiation) and physical examination (dermatomal deficits, myotomal deficits, and reflex changes).
- Perform lumbar interlaminar and transforaminal epidural steroid injections using fluoroscopy.
- Perform caudal epidural steroid injections under fluoroscopy.
- Perform lumbar medial branch blocks under fluoroscopy.
- Perform sacroiliac joint injections under fluoroscopy.
- Perform greater trochanteric bursa injections under fluoroscopy.
- Perform trigger point injections.

3. Senior Resident Clinical Objectives

▓ Demonstrate mastery of all clinical objectives listed for the junior resident rotation.

▓ Discuss the principles and indications of alternative therapeutic approaches to pain management—including acupuncture.

▓ Understand psychological interventions for chronic pain.

▓ Understand substance use disorders and detoxification options.

▓ Discuss common causes of headaches—including migraines, cluster headaches, tension headaches, cervicogenic headaches, and orofacial pain.

▓ Understand diagnostic and therapeutic intervention indications. Be able to name appropriate indications for interlaminar epidural steroid injection, transforaminal epidural steroid injection, medial branch nerve blocks, trigger point injections, piriformis and sacroiliac joint injections.

▓ Understand the anatomy of and the interventional approach to the above procedures.

▓ Describe the innervations of the medial and lateral branches of the dorsal ramus of the spinal nerve root.

▓ Correlate medial branch innervation to specific facet joint levels.

▓ Describe the innervations to the sacroiliac joints.

▓ Understand the differences between Fibromyalgia and Myofascial Pain Syndrome.

▓ Discuss causes of common neuropathic pain conditions, such as trigeminal neuralgia, phantom limb pain, complex regional pain syndrome (CRPS), and diabetic peripheral neuropathy.

▓ Discuss sickle-cell disease-related pain.

▓ Discuss common causes of chronic pelvic pain.

▓ List common entrapment neuropathies.

▓ Discuss chronic pain management in the pediatric population.

▓ Discuss chronic pain management in the geriatric population.

4. Senior Resident Skill Objectives

▧ Be able to conduct a basic evaluation of and manage a patient with chronic pain.

▧ Conduct a full pain history—include the location, radiation, duration, frequency, and pain onset. Include a pain description, alleviating and exacerbating factors and associated symptoms.

▧ Conduct a full medical, social, and surgical history. Incorporate an appropriate review of systems into a full historical examination.

▧ Conduct a full musculoskeletal and neurological physical examination—include a cranial nerve exam, stance and gait inspection examination, cervical/lumbar range of motion, upper and lower extremity manual motor testing, sensory testing and reflex examination, and appropriate provocative and nerve tension testing.

▧ Explain manual motor testing grades.

▧ Explain reflex examination scores.

▧ Provide a thorough differential diagnosis of the chief complaint.

▧ Provide a hypothesis for the level of nerve root irritation (radiculopathy) based on the history (description of pain radiation) and physical examination (dermatomal deficits, myotomal deficits, and reflex changes).

▧ Perform lumbar, thoracic, and cervical interlaminar and lumbar transforaminal epidural steroid injections using fluoroscopy.

▧ Perform caudal epidural steroid injections under fluoroscopy.

▧ Perform cervical and lumbar medial branch blocks under fluoroscopy.

▧ Perform sacroiliac joint and piriformis injections under fluoroscopy.

▧ Perform greater trochanteric bursa injections under fluoroscopy.

▧ Perform lumbar sympathetic blocks under fluoroscopy.

▧ Perform trigger point injections.

▧ Perform intra-articular injections.

▧ Perform occipital nerve blocks.

▧ Perform radiofrequency ablation or modulation of the lumbar medial branches or the sacroiliac joint.

▧ Performance of other procedures is suggested but not required: Ganglion Impar Block, Botulinum Toxin Injection, Ilioinguinal/Iliohypogastric, Pudendal Nerve Block, and Intercostal Nerve Block.

5. Key Words for Residency Inservice Examination

Anesthesia Training	PM&R Training
Neuropathic pain	Neurologic disorders: (neuropathy, plexopathy, radiculopathy)
Chronic pain: cancer: methadone	Musculoskeletal medicine: RA, OA, spondyloarthropathy, other
Somatic pain vs visceral pain	Soft tissue and orthopedic problems: acute and chronic trauma
Myofascial pain: diagnosis	Soft tissue and orthopedic problems: CRPS type II
Neuraxial opioid tolerance	Soft tissue and orthopedic problems: fibromyalgia, myofascial pain
Chronic pain: cancer: opioids	Soft tissue and orthopedic problems: spinal disorders
Celiac plexus block: indications	Soft tissue and orthopedic problems: strains, sprains, tendinitis, bursitis
Celiac plexus block: complications	Cardiovascular and other systems: cancer
Radiculopathy: steroid epidural	Rehabilitation problems and outcomes: pain, depression, substance abuse
Neuropathic pain treatment	Pharmacologic interventions: analgesics, antispasmodics, anti-inflammatories, other medications
Post-herpetic neuralgia: risk factors	Procedural/interventional: nerve blocks
CRPS II: treatment	Procedural/interventional: anesthetic injections, other procedural interventional
Stellate ganglion block; effects	
Herpes acute	

▓ FELLOWS

1. Fellows skills objectives

▓ Be able to conduct an extensive evaluation of and manage a patient with chronic pain.

▓ Conduct a full pain history: Include the location, radiation, duration, frequency, and pain onset. Include a pain description, alleviating and exacerbating factors, and associated symptoms.

▓ Conduct a full medical, social, and surgical history. Incorporate an appropriate review of systems into a full historical examination.

▓ Conduct a full musculoskeletal and neurological physical examination; include a cranial nerve exam, stance and gait inspection examination, cervical/lumbar range of motion, upper and lower extremity manual motor testing, sensory testing and reflex examination, and appropriate provocative and nerve tension testing.

▓ Explain manual motor testing grades.

▓ Explain reflex examination scores.

▓ Provide a thorough differential diagnosis of the chief complaint.

▓ Provide a hypothesis for the level of nerve root irritation (radiculopathy) based on the history (description of pain radiation) and physical examination (dermatomal deficits, myotomal deficits and reflex changes).

▓ Perform lumbar interlaminar and transforaminal epidural steroid injections using fluoroscopy.

▓ Perform caudal and epidural steroid injections under fluoroscopy.

▓ Perform cervical lumbar medial branch blocks under fluoroscopy.

▓ Perform lumbar intra-articular facet joint injections.

▓ Perform sacroiliac joint and piriformis injections under fluoroscopy.

▓ Perform greater trochanteric bursa injections under fluoroscopy.

▓ Perform trigger point injections.

▓ Perform lumbar sympathetic blocks under fluoroscopy.

▓ Perform intra-articular injections: including hip, knee, and shoulder.

▓ Perform greater and lesser occipital nerve blocks.

▓ Perform radiofrequency ablation or modulation of the cervical and lumbar medial branches.

▓ Perform radiofrequency ablation or modulation of the sacroiliac joint.

▓ Perform celiac plexus, stellate ganglion, and lumbar sympathetic blocks.

▓ Perform ilioinguinal/iliohypogastric and/or pudendal nerve blocks.

▓ Perform intercostal nerve blocks.

▓ Use botulinum toxin therapy to treat cervical dystonia, chronic headache, or myofascial pain syndrome.

▓ Perform discography and/or intradiscal electrotherapy.

▓ Perform cervical and lumbar dorsal column spinal cord stimulation trial.

▓ Perform peripheral nerve neurostimulation trial.

▓ Assist in dorsal column spinal cord stimulation implantation.

- Assist in peripheral nerve neurostimulation implantation.
- Interrogate an intrathecal pump.
- Refill an intrathecal pump.
- Assist in a baclofen intrathecal trial.
- Assist in an opioid or other analgesic intrathecal trial.
- Assist in an intrathecal pump implantation.
- Assist in an intrathecal catheter dye study.

▓ SUBSPECIALTY GOALS AND OBJECTIVES

Neuroradiology Goals and Objectives

▓ Be comfortable with the anatomy and imaging of common pain-generating degenerative spinal pathologies including: degenerative disc disease, disc herniation, facet joint pathology and cysts, spinal stenosis, spondylolysis, and spondylolisthesis.

▓ Understand the indications and contraindications of MRI and CT.

▓ Understand the advantages and limitations of MRI and CT.

▓ Learn the indications for administration of IV contrast and the possible complications.

▓ Understand the difference between T1- and T2-weighted images.

▓ Become familiar with basic neuroimaging, and identify significant findings, to include at least MR and CT of the spine and brain on a minimum of 15 CT and/or MRI studies drawn from the cervical, thoracic, and lumbar spine.

PM&R Outpatient Goals and Objectives

▓ Perform a comprehensive musculoskeletal and appropriate neuromuscular history and examination and assessment in a minimum of 15 patients, with emphasis on both structure and function.

▓ Diagnose acute and chronic pain problems based on coupling a good history with a comprehensive musculoskeletal and neurological examination.

▓ Develop multimodal treatment programs focusing on rehabilitation, functional correction, and functional restoration, including identifying and correcting the underlying body biomechanical problem, off-loading and correcting deformities or asymmetries; the assessments and treatment programs should focus on static and dynamic flexibility, strength, coordination, and agility for peripheral joint, spinal, and soft tissue pain conditions.

▓ Review the inflammatory arthridities.

▓ Review the evidence behind various physical examination provocative tests and maneuvers.

▓ Diagnose and institute treatment programs for non-spinal pain pathologies, including shoulder pain syndromes (adhesive capsulitis, impingement syndromes, rotator cuff pathology), medial and lateral epicondylitis, peripheral entrapment syndromes (carpal tunnel syndrome, ulnar neuropathy), knee and hip osteoarthritis, internal knee derangements (meniscal, ACL tears), whiplash, patellar tracking syndromes, shin splints, plantar fasciitis, and Morton's neuroma.

▓ Understand the natural history of various musculoskeletal pain disorders and be able to appropriately integrate therapeutic modalities and surgical interventions into the treatment algorithm.

SUBSPECIALTY GOALS AND OBJECTIVES (*Continued*)

PM&R Inpatient Goals and Objectives

▨ Demonstrate proficiency in the clinical evaluation and rehabilitation plan development in a minimum of 5 acute rehabilitation inpatients.

▨ Understand the role of inpatient rehabilitation in the treatment of neurological conditions such as acute spinal cord and traumatic brain injury.

▨ Understand the role of the inpatient acute rehabilitation consultation service.

▨ Understand the role of inpatients neuropsychologists, physical and occupational therapists, speech therapists, and other members of the rehabilitation team.

▨ Observe the evaluation of personal and community activities of daily living, goal planning during acute inpatient rehabilitation rounds, consultation, or FIM/team meeting.

Palliative Care Goals and Objectives

▨ Understand the clinical approach to the treatments that comprise multidisciplinary cancer pain care.

▨ Integrate the evaluation and assessment of energy level, sleep, appetite, mood, nausea, diarrhea, constipation, ambulatory status, pain, independence, and other factors into patient management planning.

▨ Understand the strategies to integrate pain management into the treatment model.

▨ Document a minimum of longitudinal involvement in the care of 20 patients.

▨ Review available interventional techniques to treat severe pain at the end of life, including: intrathecal pump implantation at the end of life, spinal and epidural neurolytic procedures, ganglioectomies, cordotomies, and other neurolytic and neuroablative procedures.

Psychiatry/Psychology Goals and Objectives

▨ Carry out a complete psychiatric history with special attention to psychiatric and pain comorbidities.

▨ Conduct a complete mental status examination on a minimum of 15 patients. (Suggest 5 completed under supervision of faculty observer.)

▨ Review frequent psychiatric and pain comorbidities, including substance related, mood, anxiety, somatiform, factitious, and personality disorders.

▨ Review the effects of pain medications on mental status.

▨ Understand the principles and techniques of the psychosocial therapies, with special attention to supportive and cognitive behavior therapies, sufficient to explain to a patient and make a referral when indicated.

SUBSPECIALTY GOALS AND OBJECTIVES (*Continued*)

Anesthesiology Goals and Objectives

- Learn the basics of airway management for sedation and general anesthesia—monitoring, mask ventilation, and securing the airway with LMA and/or endotracheal tube.
- Demonstrate competency in basic airway management, including mask ventilation in a minimum of 15 patients and endotracheal intubation in 15 patients.
- Become proficient with establishing IV access.
- Obtain IV access in a minimum of 15 patients.
- Identify superficial landmarks for placing interlaminar epidurals without the use of fluoroscopy.
- Become proficient placing lumbar and thoracic epidurals using a "blind" technique.
- Administer neuraxial analgesia to a minimum of 15 injections via a "blind" interlaminar approach.
- Learn and demonstrate competency in the management of sedation, including a direct administration of sedation to a minimum of 15 patients.

Neurology Goals and Objectives

- Review cranial nerve and head innervations.
- Review various neuromuscular junction and movement disorders.
- Review the diagnostic workup for headache, movement, and cognitive disorders.
- Review causes and presentations of dementia.
- Perform a detailed neurological examination to include at least mental status, cranial nerve, motor, sensory, reflex, cerebellar, and gait examinations in a minimum of 15 patients (suggested at least 5 are performed under the supervision of a neurologist).
- Review CT and/or MRI of the brain. (Suggested at least 2 cases with a neurologist or neuroradiologist.)

Electrodiagnostics Goals and Objectives

- Name the uses and limitations of electromyography (EMG) and nerve conduction studies (NCS).
- Name the fibers tested in quantitative sensory testing versus NCS.
- Document observation of NCS and/or EMG.
- Participate in the assessment and plan discussion in a minimum of 5 electrodiagnostic cases.

SUBSPECIALTY GOALS AND OBJECTIVES (Continued)

Pediatrics Goals and Objectives

▨ Understand the anatomic and physiologic differences that govern the rational use of analgesics in pediatric patients, including: total body water changes, fat stores, cardiac output, immaturity of the blood–brain barrier, increased renal and hepatic blood flow, and the quantity and binding ability of serum albumin and alpha-1 acid glycoprotein.

▨ Understand differences in spinal cord length, epidural content, and neurotransmitter and opiate receptors.

▨ Understand the use of specialized and developmentally appropriate pain assessment scales in acute pain assessment, including: Neonatal Infant Pain Scale (NIPS), Children's Hospital Eastern Ontario Pain Scale, FACES Pain Rating Scale, FLACC Scale (Faces/Legs/Activity/ Cry/Consolability), and N-PASS (Neonatal Pain, Agitation and Sedation Scale).

▨ Understand that the assessment of pediatric chronic pain requires a biopsychosocial perspective; include an assessment for the role of school absenteeism and family dynamics in the child's pain experience.

▨ Understand that tools for assessing chronic pediatric pain must be multidimensional.

▨ Understand the administration and use of non-opioid analgesics in pediatric patients.

▨ Understand the administration and use of opioid analgesics in oral, parenteral, and epidural form.

▨ Understand the use of oral ketamine and methadone for acute pain.

▨ Understand the application of regional analgesia techniques in the management of acute pediatric pain.

▨ Understand the role of psychology in the management of pediatric chronic pain.

▨ List the most common diagnoses in chronic pain in children and expand on their epidemiology and pathophysiology.

▨ Understand the use of interventional pain techniques in the management of chronic pain.

▨ Construct a treatment plan for chronic pain management in a pediatric patient, including the appropriate use of psychological and behavioral therapy, physical therapy, and medical therapy.

▨ Understand the challenge of managing pain in a pediatric cancer patient.

▨ Evaluate cancer-related pain.

▨ Construct a multidisciplinary pain management plan.

Suggested Formal Fellow Evaluation Systems

Patient Evaluation of Fellow	Every 1 month
Faculty Evaluation of Fellow	Every 1 month
Performance Evaluation Face-to-Face with Program Director includes case log review	Every 3 months
Faculty Evaluation by Fellow	Every 3 months
Fellow Evaluation by Resident Peer-to-Peer	Every 3 months
Fellow Evaluation by Fellow Peer-to-Peer	Every 3 months
Fellow Self-Assessment Evaluation	Every 6 months
360 Degree Evaluation Staff Evaluation of Fellow	Every 3 months
Program Evaluation by Fellow	Every 6 months
Program Evaluation by Faculty	Every 6 months
Other Evaluations: Multidisciplinary case conference, Didactics presentations, Research presentations, Obstructive structured clinical examination (OSCE)	Ongoing

Sample Pain Medicine Curriculum

A. SUGGESTED CURRICULUM OVERVIEW

First Quarter	July–September	Anesthesiology Focus: Operating Room Obstetrics/Regional
Second quarter	October–December	Palliative Care and Psychiatry Focus: Palliative Care Clinic Psychiatry Clinic
Third quarter	January–March	Neurology, Neuroradiology, and PM&R Focus: Neurology Clinic Neuroradiology PM&R Inpatient Electrodiagnostics
Fourth quarter	April–June	Pediatric and Specialty Focus: Pediatrics Elective Subspecialty

Suggested Didactics Program

B. SUGGESTED DIDACTICS PROGRAM: 1ST QUARTER

Pain Introductory Lectures
Epidemiology and Taxonomy of Pain
Anatomy & Physiology of the Pain Projection System I
Anatomy & Physiology of the Pain Projection System II
Assessment and Treatment of Pain: Note Writing Skills
Assessment and Treatment of Pain: Taking a Pain History
Assessment and Treatment of Pain: Musculoskeletal Exam: Low Back/LE
Assessment and Treatment of Pain: Musculoskeletal Exam: Neck/UE
Assessment and Treatment of Pain: Pain Measurement Techniques
Acute Pain Management: Epidural and Intrathecal Medications
Acute and Chronic Pain Management: Opioid Analgesics

Intrathecal Drug Delivery & Pump Programming
Intrathecal Drug Delivery I (Indications & Programming; Opioids)
Intrathecal Drug Delivery II (Indications & Programming; Baclofen)
Intrathecal Pump Management Challenges and Practice Session

Regional Pain Procedures & Syndromes Lectures
Epidural and Facet Injections I
Epidural and Facet Injections II
Transforaminal and Selective Nerve Root Blocks
Axial Low Back Pain: Sacroiliac Joint Pain and Joint Injections
Axial Low Back Pain: Facet-Mediated Pain
Axial Low Back Pain: Discogenic Pain
Cranial Nerve Blocks
Peripheral Nerve Blocks and Ablation
Prevention, Recognition and Management of Local Anesthetic, Contrast and Steroid Overdose
Sympathetic Blocks

Epidemiology Lectures I and II
Epidemiology & Biostatistics I
Epidemiology & Biostatistics II

PM&R Physical Examination Practice Sessions
PM&R Physical Examination Practice Session: Cervical/UE
PM&R Physical Examination Practice Session: Lumbar/LE

C. SUGGESTED DIDACTICS PROGRAM: 2ND QUARTER

Specialty Lectures: Teaching Skills
Teaching Fellows to Teach

Palliative Care Lectures
Geriatric Issues in Pain Management
Ethics of Pain & Palliative Care
Palliative Care Principles I
Palliative Care Principles II
Management of Opioid-Induced Constipation & Nausea
Neurolytic & Interventional Options for End-of-Life Pain Management

Research Study Design
Research Study Design I
Research Study Design II

Pain Practice Design
Organization of a Pain Practice

Psychiatry Lectures
Substance Abuse
Personality Disorders in Pain
Depression in the Context of Chronic Pain
Anxiety in the Context of Chronic Pain
Principles of Addiction Medicine
Psychological Modalities & Behavioral Therapies with Cultural and Cross-Cultural Considerations

SCS Simulation/Cadaver Workshop
Spinal Cord Stimulation Simulation and/or Cadaveric Workshop

D. SUGGESTED DIDACTICS PROGRAM: 3RD QUARTER

Electrodiagnostics Principles
Electrodiagnostics Principles

Neurology Lectures
Neuropathic Pain Syndromes
Peripheral Neuropathies
Complex Regional Pain Syndrome (CRPS)
Tension & Cluster Headaches
Migraine Headaches
Facial Pain Syndromes

Neuroradiology and Surgical Lectures
Minimally Invasive Cervical Spine Surgery
Minimally Invasive Lumbar Spine Surgery
MRI Neuroradiology Review I
MRI Neuroradiology Review II
Total Disc Replacement

PM&R Lectures
Myofascial Pain Syndrome
Fibromyalgia
Joint & Bursal Injections
Acupuncture in Pain Medicine
The Physical Modalities in Pain Medicine
Central Pain Syndromes—SCI, Stroke Pain & Amputation-Related Pains

E. SUGGESTED DIDACTICS PROGRAM: 4TH QUARTER

Pediatrics Lectures
Assessment of Pain in Children
Psychosocial Pediatric Pain Management

Specialty Lectures: Systems Management
Patient and Provider Safety
Pain Quality Improvement & Utilization Review
Billing & Coding: E&M Training
Pharmacy Medicare Part D Update

Specialty Lectures: Special Pain Syndromes
Visceral and Urogenital Pain
Pelvic Pain
Pain in the Pregnant Patient
Osteoarthritis and Inflammatory Arthritis

Specialty Lectures: Adjunctive Medications
Antispasmodic and Non-Steroidal Anti-Inflammatory Agents
Anti-Depressants for Pain: TCAs and SNRIs
Anti-Convulsants for Pain: Calcium and Calcium/Sodium Blockers
NMDA-Antagonists: Methadone and Ketamine Safety

Cognitive Objectives

Month 1

- Understand the processes resulting in noxious-stimulus induced pain, including transduction, transmission, modulation, and perception.
- Name stimuli that peripheral nociceptors respond to.
- Delineate the anatomic organization of the dorsal horn.
- Name the terminations for unmyelinated C fibers and large myelinated fibers.
- Understand the differential input to the wide dynamic range and nociceptive specific second-order neurons.
- Understand the two main signaling channels in the somatosensory system: the anterolateral and dorsal column-medial lemniscal system; understand their unique projections.
- Understand the multitude of locations where derangements can occur resulting in the generation of chronic pain.
- Name the key excitatory neurotransmitters in the somatosensory system and name the four key excitatory amino acid receptors.
- Name the key inhibitory neurotransmitters.
- Name important excitatory and inhibitory neuropeptides in the somatosensory system.
- Define: Analgesia, anesthesia, anesthesia dolorosa, central pain, chronic pain, deafferentation pain, dysesthesia, hyperalgesia, hyperesthesia, hyperpathia, hypoalgesia, hypoesthesia, neuralgia, neuritis, neurogenic pain, neuropathic pain, nociceptive pain, somatic pain, visceral pain, paresthesia, radicular pain, radiculopathy, referred pain and suffering.
- Name unidimensional and multidimensional pain assessment scales.
- Understand which scales are better used in the pediatric population and which are better employed in the geriatric population.
- Understand that healthcare professionals' judgment cannot be substituted for a patient's self-report of his or her pain.
- List the key domains for the psychological evaluation of pain. Understand the importance of personality assessment and what screening tool is usually employed.
- Name the uses and limitations of EMG and NCS.
- Name the fibers tested in quantitative sensory testing versus nerve conduction studies.
- Be comfortable with the anatomy of and imaging of common pain-generating degenerative spinal pathologies including: degenerative disc disease, disc herniation, facet joint pathology and cysts, spinal stenosis, spondylolysis and spondylolisthesis. Understand when MRI is preferred over CT imaging; discuss when gadolinium is used.

Month 2

- Explain the epidemiology of pain and its economic impact.
- Understand how to determine impairment, including use of the Functional Capacity Examination and Work Capacity Evaluation.
- Understand that the vast majority of accommodations or work-site modifications cost less than $300.
- Understand major, minor, and short-acting opioid use in pain management.
- Recite the properties of meperidine, morphine, oxycodone, hydromorphone, methadone, hydrocodone, codeine, tramadol, propoxyphene, and fentanyl.
- Recite conversion ratios among opioids.
- Understand adverse effects of opioid therapy, including addiction.
- Define addiction, physical dependence, pseudoaddiction, and tolerance.
- Name the most common illegal drug-related behaviors (aberrant behaviors suggestive of prescription drug abuse).
- Screen for subtle signs of opioid abuse, including a focus on opioids and avoidance of other treatment modalities, early refills, escalating doses, multiple telephone calls, a pattern of prescription problems and use of supplemental opioid sources.
- State the *DSM-IV* Criteria for Substance Dependence and Substance Abuse.
- List the 3 types of urine drug toxicity screens and their mechanism of action.
- Understand the duration of a positive urine test for major abused substances; name limitations with testing. Be aware of other ways to evaluate suspicious patients, including pill counting and the California Patient Activity Report.
- Name the most common side effects of opioid therapy and which effects do not acquire tolerance over time.
- Name the most useful agents to treat opioid-induced constipation.
- Name the multiple treatment outcomes that should be assessed with opioid therapy.
- Name standardized instruments for subjective pain reduction, evidence of improved functional status and quality of life.
- List examples of DEA Schedule I through V controlled substances and a description of the criteria for each schedule.
- Name the signs of opioid withdrawal and intoxication (overnarcotization).
- Name the side effects of Narcan use; be able to set up an infusion.

Month 3

▦ Name the safer opioids to use in: renal dysfunction, pregnancy, lactation, liver failure, and in the geriatric population.

▦ Name the two phases of drug metabolism.

▦ Understand metabolic considerations for morphine, codeine, and hydrocodone.

▦ Name inhibitors and inducers of the P2D6 and 3A4 enzyme systems.

▦ Name metabolites with greater analgesia than their parent compounds.

▦ Understand the use of adjunctive analgesic medications, including membrane stabilizers, antidepressants, NSAIDs, and antispasmodics.

▦ Recite the pathway for formation of prostaglandins.

▦ Review NSAID toxicity.

▦ Explain what receptors are targeted with adjuvant medication use.

▦ List limitations and warnings for TCAs, SNRIs, mood stabilizers, neuroleptics, and others.

▦ Name potential neuropathic receptor/medication targets, including TCA, SNRI, NMDA antagonism, sodium channel blockade, substance P inhibition, alpha-2 agonism, opioids, calcium channel blockade, and mixed sodium channel/calcium channel blockade.

▦ Understand the use of titration schedules for neuropathic medications.

▦ State the mechanism of action for: benzodiazepines, baclofen, tizanidine, dantrolene, botulinum toxin, cyclobenzaprine, carisoprodol, and methocarbamol.

▦ List approved radiocontrast agents for spinal injections.

▦ Name potential adverse reactions associated with contrast agents as well as pre-treatment regimens.

▦ Discuss what determines the potency, speed of onset, and duration of action for local anesthetics; list the differential properties for lidocaine and bupivacaine.

▦ Name adverse reactions associated with local anesthetics.

▦ Name potential adverse reactions associated with corticosteroids.

▦ Discuss clinical applications to botulinum toxin therapy, including cervical dystonia, TMJ disorder, headaches, whiplash injury, hemifacial pain, LBP, myofascial pain, and piriformis syndrome.

▦ Understand the potential independent analgesic properties of botulinum toxin.

Month 4

▦ Understand the role of differential neural blockade for diagnosis, including the frequency of placebo responders.

▦ Be aware of neurosurgical procedures for the treatment of intractable pain, including: spinal dorsal rhizotomy, dorsal root ganglionectomy, facet denervation, peripheral neurectomy, sympathectomy, lesions of the dorsal root entry zone, commissural myelotomy, anterolateral cordotomy, and intracranial ablative procedures.

▦ Discuss the principles and indications of physical medicine and rehabilitation (PM&R) approaches to pain management, including the use of occupational and physical therapy programs, orthotics use, and the use of the physical modalities.

▦ State the basic indications for heating versus cold modalities.

▦ State precautions for the use of ultrasound as a deep heating modality.

▦ Name contraindications to chiropractic therapy.

▦ Discuss the principles and indications of alternative therapeutic approaches to pain management, including acupuncture.

▦ Name mechanisms of action for electroacupuncture therapy.

▦ State the contraindications to acupuncture therapy.

▦ Understand pain and its relation to psychosocial issues.

▦ Understand pain and its relation to depression and other psychiatric illnesses.

▦ Understand psychological interventions for chronic pain, including: operant interventions, relaxation interventions, biofeedback, cognitive–behavioral interventions, and hypnosis.

▦ Understand substance use disorders (abuse, addiction, misuse, physical dependence, and psychological dependence) and detoxification options.

▦ State the approximate percentage of substance abuse in the United States.

▦ Name the most common illicit substance, most common abused substance, and the most common abused pain medication.

▦ State the approximate success rates of: 5-day simple detoxification versus 6-month detoxification.

▦ List signs and symptoms of sedative-hypnotic withdrawal.

Month 5

▧ Understand pain in the Emergency Department.

▧ Understand that postoperative pain results from peripheral and central sensitization. Describe the concept of preemptive analgesia.

▧ Describe the safety of patient-controlled analgesia (PCA).

▧ List limitations to the use of the PCA, including younger age and patients with mental and physical handicaps.

▧ List common adult and pediatric PCA doses.

▧ Specify the indications for the use of a basal infusion.

▧ Differentiate the extent of (hydro-) versus lipophilicity of fentanyl and morphine with respect to onset of action, duration of action, and side effects with respect to intrathecal and/or epidural opioid use.

▧ List factors that may contribute to the development of respiratory depression after intrathecal opioid administration.

▧ List potential benefits to perioperative epidural use (when compared with systemic opioids).

▧ List common side effects of epidural opioids.

▧ State basic anatomic and physiologic differences in pediatric patients.

▧ Name developmentally appropriate pain assessment scales for use in infants and children respectively.

▧ Review the use of aspirin, epidural analgesia, intravenous and epidural PCA analgesia in the pediatric population.

▧ Describe the U.S. Food and Drug Administration Pregnancy Category System (categories A, B, C, D, and X) and list common drugs in each category. List drugs to absolutely avoid during pregnancy.

▧ Name drugs associated with reversible oligohydramnios and cleft lip/palate.

▧ List drugs safe for use in lactation. Name properties of safe drugs, including molecular weight, ionization, lipid solubility, and protein binding ability.

▧ List drugs to absolutely avoid during lactation.

▧ Review pain control in the critically ill patient.

Month 6

- Explain the pathophysiology of migraine headaches.
- List migraine abortive and prophylactic treatment medications.
- Explain the pathophysiology and treatment of cluster headaches.
- Discuss the diagnostic features of tension-type headaches.
- List abortive and prophylactic medications for tension-type headaches.
- Name the signs and symptoms, pathophysiology, and initial therapy of postdural puncture headache (PDPH).
- State the percentage of PDPHs that resolves spontaneously in five days.
- Discuss the effects of caffeine, theophylline, and the epidural blood patch.
- Explain the mechanism of cervicogenic headache.
- Explain the diagnosis and management of trigeminal neuralgia and temporomandibular disorder.
- Define acute and chronic back pain; define axial and radicular pain.
- Explain common causes of mechanical low back pain, including muscle strain, discogenic disease, vertebral fracture (compression), myofascial pain syndrome, facet arthropathy (lumbar spondylosis), hip osteoarthritis, and sacroiliac dysfunction.
- Review the anatomy and innervation of spinal ligaments, paraspinal musculature, vertebral body periosteum, the intervertebral disc and the facet joints with special attention to the sinuvertebral nerve and the medial branch nerve of the posterior primary ramus.
- List the indications and controversy surrounding the surgical treatment of LBP, including: decompression, fusion, and disc replacement.
- Understand diagnostic and therapeutic intervention indications, anatomy, and approach for interlaminar epidural steroid injection, transforaminal epidural steroid injection, medial branch nerve blocks, trigger point injections, piriformis and sacroiliac joint injections.
- Describe the innervations of the medial and lateral branches of the dorsal ramus of the spinal nerve root and correlate medial branch innervation to specific facet joint levels.
- Describe the innervations to the sacroiliac joints.
- Understand the differences between fibromyalgia and myofascial pain.
- Review the evidence on trigger point injections for myofascial pain.
- List the American College of Rheumatology Diagnostic Criteria for Fibromyalgia.
- Describe the central pathology, associated conductions, and the management of fibromyalgia.

Month 7

- List the principal clinical components of CRPS I and II. Name diagnostic tests useful in the workup. State bone-scan changes in CRPS.
- Understand the use of guanethidine and phentolamine infusions.
- Name a variety of treatment modalities for CRPS.
- Discuss the epidemiology, natural history, and treatment of herpes zoster, and the pathophysiology and pharmacologic treatment of post-herpetic neuralgia. Name the location of latency of the herpes zoster virus. State the typical rash duration. Name risk factors for post-herpetic neuralgia (PHN). Explain the role of interventional pain management in the treatment of PHN.
- Define phantom sensation, telescoping, phantom pain, and stump pain. State their incidences. Review phantom phenomena post-mastectomy.
- Discuss the most common causes of central pain.
- Discuss the clinical presentation of pain in the spinal cord injury patient.
- Explain visceral pain and viscerosomatic convergence.
- List stimuli that can induce visceral pain.
- Discuss the most common causes of chronic pelvic pain.
- State the molecular event that underlies the manifestations of sickle cell disease. List factors that can precipitate a sickle cell crisis; discuss the acute management of sickle cell crisis.
- State central mechanisms that can explain neuropathic pain. Name metabolic, nutritional, toxic, genetic, and infectious etiologies of painful peripheral neuropathies.
- Define Charcot joint.
- Discuss the use of NCS/EMG and quantitative sensory testing (QST) in the workup of painful peripheral neuropathy.
- Explain the pathology, symptoms, risk factors, and treatment of: carpal tunnel syndrome, cubital tunnel syndrome, thoracic outlet syndrome, meralgia paresthetica, and tarsal tunnel syndrome.
- State the most common causes of chronic pain in the pediatric population. State the gender preference of CRPS in the pediatric population.
- Discuss the assessment of pain in the geriatric population.
- State the effects of untreated pain in the elderly.
- List common pain behaviors in cognitively impaired elderly persons.
- List changes in physiology, including metabolic ones, in geriatric medicine.
- Name medications that should be avoided in the geriatric population.

Month 8

- Explain the gate control theory.
- List the criteria for appropriate patient selection for spinal cord stimulation.
- Discuss the use of SCS for postlaminectomy syndrome, CRPS, and peripheral ischemia and angina.
- State the most common SCS complication.
- Name the final lead placement location for cervical and lumbar stimulation.
- List intraspinally administered drugs in the treatment of intractable pain. List FDA-approved drugs for this purpose. List the most widely recognized side effects of intraspinal narcotics.
- Discuss complications of intrathecal pump implantation use, including: infection, infusion of contaminated drug, hardware erosion, pump failure, catheter problems, and seroma.
- State the innervation to the intervertebral disc. Describe symptoms of discogenic pain. State indications for lumbar discography. Discuss the use of manometric discography. List the potential and most common complications of discography.
- Name diagnostic criteria for intradiscal electrotherapies (IDET, RF, discTRODE RF annuloplasty and disc biacuplasty). Discuss possible mechanisms of action for intradiscal electrotherapies.
- Review conservative management of osteoporosis and compression fractures. Discuss indications and contraindications for vertebroplasty and kyphoplasty. Review the advantages and disadvantages of each.
- State the maximum permissible dose of radiation: annual whole-body dose limit. State the annual maximum permissible fetal dose.
- Define ALARA in radiology.
- Discuss distance of the X-ray tube and image intensifier; discuss collimation, live fluoroscopy, freeze frames, and magnification in minimizing patient exposure. State the thickness and shielding of lead aprons.
- List patients at a greater risk of a severe reaction to radiologic contrast.
- Explain the World Health Organization's ladder approach to cancer pain treatment.
- Review the use of corticosteroids as adjunctive analgesics in the cancer pain population.
- Delineate palliative and hospice care.
- List causes of neuropathic pain in cancer and at the end of life.
- Review pain syndromes in end-of-life cardiovascular disease, cirrhosis, debility, renal disease, neuromuscular disorders, and pulmonary disease.
- Define air hunger and state its treatment modalities.
- Define the principle of double effect.

Month 9

- State indications for neurolytic celiac plexus block. Discuss the technique and complications from celiac plexus blocks.
- Discuss the utility and technique of superior hypogastric and ganglion impar sympathetic blocks.
- Discuss how alcohol and phenol cause neurolysis (mechanisms of action).
- Compare alcohol and phenol with respect to solubility in body fluids, pain on injection, and baricity to CSF. Discuss patient positioning for neurolysis depending on the use of alcohol and phenol in the CSF.
- State concentrations needed for sensory block and motor block for both alcohol and phenol.
- List indications and complications for neuraxial neurolytic block.
- List agents that can potentiate local anesthetics.
- Review systemic effects of lidocaine and other local anesthetics and the relative potencies for central nervous system and cardiovascular system toxicities.
- List the structures the spinal needle passes through before reaching the subarachnoid space.
- State the most common locale for: the caudal tip of the spinal cord, the cauda equine, and the epidural space.
- Review factors that influence block height and duration of block in spinal anesthesia; review physiologic effects of spinal anesthesia.
- List the contents of the epidural space.
- Review factors affecting the spread within the epidural space.
- Discuss the diagnosis of spinal epidural hematoma and epidural abscess.
- Review combined spinal-epidural techniques.
- Discuss the indications and technique of caudal epidural block.
- List the frequency of local anesthetic-induced seizures in adults between various interventional techniques.
- Review the techniques of lysis of epidural adhesions.
- State the indications and landmarks for glossopharyngeal nerve block. List complications, including the most common inadvertent nerve blocks and their physical manifestations (vagus, hypoglossal, and accessory).
- Describe the result of bilateral glossopharyngeal nerve block.
- List the indications and complications of phrenic nerve block.
- Draw the 4 branches of the superficial cervical plexus.
- Describe the advantages to carotid artery surgery performed under combined superficial and deep cervical plexus block. Discuss the technique and complications of both the superficial and deep blocks.
- Review the anatomy of the greater occipital nerve, greater occipital protuberance, occipital artery, and lesser occipital nerve.

Month 10

- Draw the brachial plexus and list the motor innervations of the upper extremity.
- Review supra- and infraclavicular approaches to brachial plexus blocks, including the interscalene, supraclavicular and axillary/infraclavicular techniques. Name the safest technique. Name the technique with the highest incidence of pneumothorax. Name the technique with the highest incidence of phrenic nerve block. Name the technique associated with the highest incidence of intravascular injection of local anesthetics.
- Discuss the roots frequently missed with an interscalene block. Draw a cross-section of the axillary sheath for axillary/infraclavicular brachial plexus block with quadrants for the major nerves, humerus, artery, and vein.
- State the indication for surgical axillary brachial plexus block (arm surgery below the elbow, including wrist and hand).
- State the anatomic landmarks for radial, ulnar, and median nerve blocks at both the level of the elbow and the wrist.
- Draw intercostal nerve anatomy; state complications of intercostal blocks.
- List the means through which paravertebral blocks can provide anesthesia to several dermatomes.
- State the indications for suprascapular, ilioinguinal, and iliohypogastric nerve blocks.
- State the anatomic landmarks for ilioinguinal, iliohypogastric, obturator, genitofemoral, lateral femoral cutaneous, femoral and sciatic nerve blocks.
- Review the indications and technique of lumbar plexus block.
- Name the only cutaneous branch of the posterior division of the femoral nerve.
- List the two divisions of the sciatic nerve: their supplied muscles and the action of those muscles.
- Review the posterior (classic) approach and popliteal fossa approach to sciatic nerve block.
- State the anatomic landmarks for tibial, saphenous, sural, superficial peroneal, and deep peroneal ankle blocks.
- Name the anatomic location of the cervicothoracic ganglion (stellate). Discuss the risk of local anesthetic injection into the vertebral artery; discuss the significance of the appearance of Horner's Syndrome.
- Name the anatomic location of the lumbar sympathetic ganglia. Name the signs, symptoms, and tests that signify complete sympathetic blockade.
- Review complications of neuraxial and peripheral blocks.
- Recite the ASRA Guidelines on anticoagulants and neuraxial anesthesia/analgesia.

References

Abdi S, et al. A new and easy technique to block the stellate ganglion. *Pain Physician.* 2004;7:327–331.

ACOG Practice Bulletin No. 51. Chronic pelvic pain. *Obstet Gynecol.* 2004 Mar;103(3):589–605.

Albazaz R, et al. Complex regional pain syndrome: A review. *Ann Vasc Surg.* 2008 Mar;22(2):297–306.

Benzon, et al. Comparison of the particle sizes of different steroids and the effect of dilution. *Anesthesiology* 2007;106:331–338.

Botelho RJ, Sitzman BT. Pharmacology for the interventional pain physician. *Essentials of Pain Medicine* (Chap. 19, 3rd edition).

Chahl LA. Opioids—mechanism of action. *Aust Prescr.* 1996;19:63–65.

Cone EJ, Heit HA, et al. Evidence of morphine metabolism to hydromorphone in pain patients chronically treated with morphine. *J Anal Toxicol.* 2006; 30:1–5.

Fardon, et al. Nomenclature and Classification of Lumbar Disc Pathology. *Spine.* 2001;(26):E93–E113.

Hasslesstrom J, Sawe J. Morphine pharmacokinetics and metabolism in humans. Enterohepatic cycling and relative contribution of metabolites to active opioid concentrations. *Clin Pharmacokinetics* 2001;40:344–354.

Headache Classification Subcommittee of the International Headache Society. The International Classification of Headache Disorders (2nd edition). *Cephalalgia* 2004;(24 Suppl 1):9–160.

Inturrisi CE. Clinical pharmacology of opioids for pain. *Clin J Pain.* 2002;18: S3–13.

Modesto-Lowe V. Methadone deaths: risk factors in pain and addicted populations. *J Gen Intern Med.* 2010 April;25(4):305–309.

Moeller K, Lee K, Kissack J. Urine drug screening: practical guide for clinicians. *Mayo Clinic Proc.* 2008;83:66–76.

Neal JM, Bernards CM, Butterworth JF. ASRA practice advisory on local anesthetic systemic toxicity. *Reg Anesth Pain Med.* 2010 Mar-Apr;35(2):152–161.

Pham, P, et al. Pain Management in Patients with Chronic Kidney Disease. *NDT Plus.* 2009;2:111–118.

Reisfield GM, Salazar E, Bertholf RL. Rational use and interpretation of urine drug testing in chronic opioid therapy. *Ann Clin Lab Sci.* 2007;37:301–314.

Sandoval JA. Oral methadone for chronic noncancer pain: A systematic literature review of reasons for administration, prescription patterns, effectiveness, and side effects. *Clin J Pain* 2005 Nov-Dec;21(6):503–512.

Shapiro LE, Shear NH. Drug interactions:Proteins, pumps, and P-450s. *J Am Acad Dermatol* 2002;47:467–484.

Smith G, Stubbins MJ, Harries LW, Wolf CR. (1999). Molecular genetics of the human cytochrome P450 monooxygenase superfamily. *Xenobiotica* 28(12): 1129–1165.

Stoelting RK. *Pharmacology, Physiology and Anesthetic Practice.* 2nd Ed. Lippincott Williams and Wilkins, Baltimore, 1991.

Wasan AD, Michna E, et al. Interpreting urine drug tests: Prevalence of morphine metabolism to hydromorphone in chronic pain patients treated with morphine. *Pain Med* 2008;9:918–923.

Waxman SG (2010). Chapter 8. Cranial Nerves and Pathways. In S.G. Waxman (Ed.), *Clinical Neuroanatomy*, 26e. Retrieved November 11, 2012 from http://www.accessmedicine.com/content.aspx?aID=5272646

West R, Crews B, et al. Anomalous observations of codeine in patients on morphine. *Therapeutic Drug Monitoring* 2009;31:776–778.

West R, West C, et al. Anomalous observations of hydrocodone in patients on oxycodone. *Clinica Chimica Acta* 2011;412:29-32.

www.PDR.net

http://www.fda.gov/Drugs/DrugSafety/default.htm

http://www.who.int/maternal_child_adolescent/documents/55732/en

http://www.perinatology.com/exposures/druglist.htm

http://professional.medtronic.com/wcm/groups/mdtcom_sg/@mdt/@neuro/documents/documents/pump-indc-refmanl.pdf